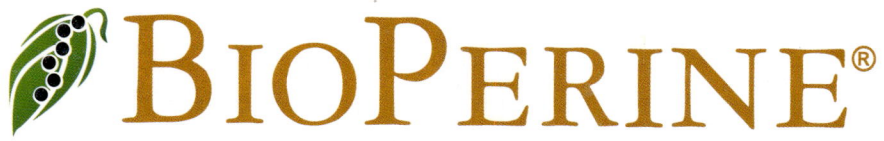

BioPerine®

Nature's Own Supernutrient

US 5,536,506; US 5,744,161; US 5,972,382; US 6,054,585; CA 2247467; EP 0810868; JP 3953513

Bioavailability Enhancer • Thermonutrient

Edited by:

Muhammed Majeed, Ph.D.

Kalyanam Nagabhushanam, Ph.D.

Authors:

Muhammed Majeed, Ph.D.

Kalyanam Nagabhushanam, Ph.D.

Lakshmi Mundkur, Ph.D.

Smitha Thazhathidath, M. Sc.

Mahesh Paschapur, M. Pharm.

T. Samuel Manoharan, Ph.D.

First Printing
NutriScience Publishers, LLC
East Windsor, New Jersey, The United States of America

Disclaimer

The information contained in this book, **BioPerine®—Nature's Own Supernutrient, Bioavailability Enhancer and Thermonutrient,** is intended to provide helpful and informative material for scientific and educational purposes only. It is not intended to diagnose, treat, cure, or prevent any health problem or condition. It is not designed, in whole or in part, as an advice for self-diagnosis or self-treatment; nor is intended to serve as a replacement for professional medical advice.

NutriScience Publishers, LLC
20 Lake Drive, East Windsor
New Jersey, 08520
The United States of America

Copyright © 2017 NutriScience Publishers, LLC

All rights reserved, including the right of reproduction in whole or in part in any form.

NutriScience Publishers, LLC First Edition 2017
ISBN: 978-0-9883209-2-5

Preface

"All that man needs for good health and healing can be found in nature; it is the job of science to find it."

—Paracelsus (1493 – 1541)

'Our Innovation Is Your Answer®', the tagline of Sabinsa, underscores our diligent dedication and tireless quest to bring in the enormous knowledge of Ayurveda, the Indian traditional system of medicine, to help you live longer, happier and healthier!

Our journey to integrate ancient wisdom from India with the Western world began in late 1980s when we introduced Ayurveda to the Americans as a complete system with holistic healing approach.

Time and again, it is proven that body's nutritional need is majorly taken care by the food that we eat every day. However, in recent years, researchers have observed an astounding link between lifestyle, individual health and quality of life. Unhealthy lifestyle has sparked an epidemic of chronic diseases, which are the major causes of global health concerns. According to World Health Organization report, ~60% of factors that considerably influence overall health and wellness are correlated to changing lifestyle.

Additionally, in the current day rush, normal life is no more normal as people are giving up the idea of balanced nutrition. Consequently, there exists a wide gap between proper nutrient intake and optimal health, which is very essential, given the reducing affordability to manage various health conditions, both in terms of time and money.

However, in recent decade, people have started to understand the difference between just 'being healthy' and 'feeling healthy', as they began to realize the significance of health and lifestyle, and role of nutritional supplements, which could help bring one closer to the state of 'healthy life'.

Several quality natural products from Sami-Sabinsa Group have made noteworthy impact in nutrition and healthcare market. One such product is **BioPerine®**, a patented extract (standardized to minimum 95% piperine) obtained from the fruits of Piper nigrum (Black pepper). This revered spice is popularly termed as "King of Spices" due to its supreme and unique position across the globe.

*"**Pepper is the bride around which everyone dances**" these lines by Jacob Hustaert, Governor of Sri Lanka for Dutch East India Company in 1664, further corroborate the fact that pepper has been influential across the world.*

It is the indefatigable and concerted effort of the research team of Sami-Sabinsa Group from past couple of decades that has added scientific credentials to piperine, which includes 'bioavailability enhancement' and 'thermonutrient' properties, along with biological and pharmacological effects both in animals and humans.

Though our earlier book on BioPerine® did discuss about various aspects of piperine, we have highlighted recent developments and research findings pertaining to historical background, chemistry, bioenhancement and thermonutrient mechanism, metabolism, bioavailability enhancement of various xenobiotics, and pharmacological and safety profile of piperine in detail in the present book.

As more and more people around the world are recognizing the importance of being hale and hearty, nature-based molecules are getting significant attention in global health debates as they hold promise for their holistic approach to health and nourishment, while addressing modern day health challenges.

Going forward, we expect that mainstream medicine would be more open to alternative/complementary medicine, to form an integrative healthcare system, to address the physical and emotional well being of individuals. And we also hope that in coming days research on traditional herbal medicine will play a critical role in global health that would contemplate what lay ahead for the human health and wellness.

It is our firm belief that this book would rekindle our interest in holistic benefits of traditional medicines all over again, augmented with the flavor of science.

We are grateful to all those scientists whose constant efforts during last couple of decades unravelled the mystery behind the distinctive ability of this phytochemical. We also congratulate our scientists from Sami-Sabinsa who have dedicatedly worked to help better understand diverse benefits of this supernutrient.

We wish you and your beloved ones the very health and happiness, today and everyday!

- Muhammed Majeed, Ph.D.
- Kalyanam Nagabhushanam, Ph.D.

ABOUT THE EDITORS

Muhammed Majeed, Ph.D.

Dr. Muhammed Majeed holds a doctorate (1986) in Industrial Pharmacy from St. John's University, New York. He has over 14 years of pharmaceutical research experience in the United States with leading pharma companies, such as Pfizer Inc., Carter-Wallace and Paco Research.

Subsequent to the formation of his company, Sabinsa Corporation in 1988, he has pursued his interest in phytochemistry and pharmaceutical sciences. He has led a team of scientists, both in India & the USA, and obtained 157+ USA and International patents so far. He is aggressively pursuing his interest in natural products and continues to develop new products for the USA and International markets.

Kalyanam Nagabhushanam, Ph.D.

Dr. Kalyanam Nagabhushanam is the President of Sami-Sabinsa Group R&D. His research interests are in synthetic methodology, chiral chemistry and natural products. He obtained his M.Sc. in Chemistry from University of Madras and Ph.D. from Baylor, Texas. After a further two-year post-doctoral studies in the USA on chiral chemistry and chiro-optical methods, he returned to India to work with IPCL (now part of Reliance group), Ciba-Geigy (now known as Novartis) and SPIC Pharma. He has been with Sabinsa for the last 17 years. Dr. Kalyanam's primary reponsibilities at Sabinsa include development of new products and exploration of new business areas.

ABOUT THE AUTHORS

Lakshmi Mundkur, Ph.D.

Dr. Lakshmi Mundkur obtained her M. Sc. and Ph.D. in Biotechnology, specializing in Immunology from Madurai Kamaraj University, Madurai. She started her career with Lupin Chemicals Ltd. (India) and moved on to Wockhardt Research Centre (India), Novartis Healthcare (India) and Thrombosis Research Institute (India) during her 20 years of experience in pharma and drug discovery research. Her research interests include immunology, molecular biology and mechanism of action of natural products. Presently, she is the Vice President of Biological Research at Sami Labs. Her major responsibilities at Sami-Sabinsa are to explore the biological efficacy and mechanism of action of new products.

Smitha Thazhathidath, M. Sc.

Smitha Thazhathidath holds Master's degree in Biochemistry from Bangalore University, Bangalore and has been with Sami Labs for over 9 years. She holds the position of Senior Executive – Technical Support, which works as an important bridge between the global marketing/business development team and the R&D team. She provides overall technical and techno-marketing support to all business development teams of Sami-Sabinsa Group.

Mahesh Paschapur, M. Pharm.

Mahesh Paschapur has done his M. Pharm. from K. L. E. S's College of Pharmacy, Belagavi. Presently, he is a part of Technical Support Department of Sami Labs, which acts as an interface between R&D division and business development/ marketing team. He is majorly involved in supporting Sami-Sabinsa representatives and clients with scientific content writing as well as various techno-marketing write-ups. He has 6 years of research experience in the field of neuropharmacology, affective disorders, treatment-resistant depression and fibrosis. Prior to joining Sami Labs he was associated with Biocon-Bristol-Myers Squibb Research Center, Bangalore.

T. Samuel Manoharan, Ph.D.

Dr. T. Samuel Manoharan is a Principal Scientist and General Manager, Synthetic Chemistry and Biocatalysis Division, Sami Labs. He has done his Ph.D. in Organic Chemistry at Indian Institute of Science, Bangalore (1985) followed by post-doctoral training in Canada at University of Alberta, Edmonton (1986–1989) and Brock University, St. Catharines, Ontario (1989–1991). He worked as a Senior Scientist and Manager (R&D) at Southern Petrochemical Industries Corporation Ltd., Tuticorin between 1991–2003 before joining Sami Labs in 2004.

© NutriScience Publishers, LLC. 2017

CONTENTS

BioPerine®—Nature's Own Supernutrient, Bioavailability Enhancer and Thermonutrient

01	Pepper...the Botanic Helen of Troy	1
02	Mechanism of Bioenhancement by Piperine	15
03	Bioavailability Enhancer	35
04	Piperine and its Health Benefits	71
	Antioxidant Activity	72
	Anti-inflammatory Activity	80
	Anticancer Activity	91
	Management of Metabolic Syndrome	106
	Neuropharmacological Effects	129
	Influence on Digestive System	149
	Respiratory Health Support	154
	Ergogenic Effects	161
05	Metabolism of Piperine	171
06	Long-term Safety of Piperine	177
	BioPerine®: Reconciling Traditional Knowledge with Modern Benefits	190
	BioPerine® and GRAS Status	191
	Sabinsa's Intellectual Property Portfolio on BioPerine®	193
	Analytical Profile	195
	Conclusion	205
	References	209
	Glossary	229

© NutriScience Publishers, LLC. 2017

Chapter 1
Pepper...
the Botanic Helen of Troy

*"**Pepper...the Botanic Helen of Troy**"*, exclaimed Marjorie Shaffer, a science writer and editor at New York University School of Medicine, in her recent book entitled "Pepper—A History of the World's Most Influential Spice." These introductory lines would connote our long-standing obsession with spices, pepper, in particular.

She goes on to proclaim that pepper launched a thousand ships carrying it in trade just like the beautiful countenance of Helen launched thousand ships in war. This comparison is very apt, as it is the passion for this exotic spice that instigated the new era of global trade, and in turn the world history (Shaffer, 2013).

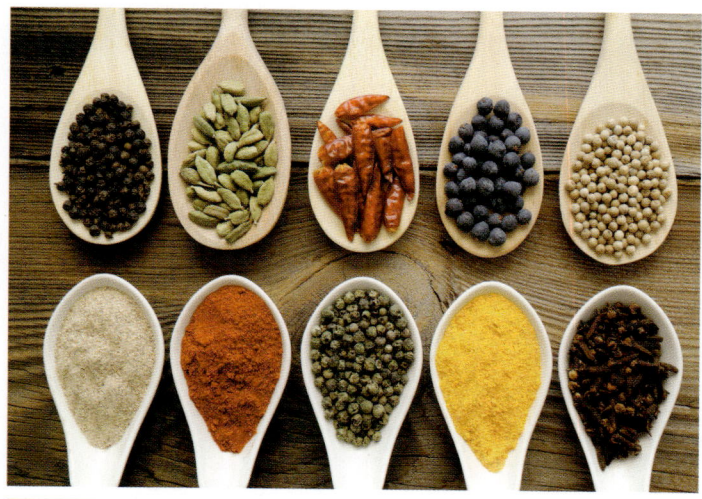

Today, we clearly distinguish herbs from spices; however, during olden days all aromatic plant products were known as herbs. While small aromatic, temperate leafy plants, such as coriander, mint and basil are categorized as herbs, which is derived from the Latin word *"herba"*—meaning 'grass' or 'green stalks', spices is the term used to denote dried pieces obtained from flowers, fruits, buds, seeds, bark and rhizome of specific tropical plants, such as peppercorns, cloves and cinnamon. The word 'spice' is derived from the Latin word *"species"*—meaning 'specific kind'. However, during Roman era, the term 'spice' was designated to valuable articles, and also to indicate certain dutiable goods (Narsimhan, 2009).

Spice, in general, has been defined as a strongly flavored or aromatic substance of vegetable origin, commonly used as a condiment. In ancient times, spices were as precious as gold; and as significant as medicines.

The history of spice is almost as old as human civilization, and India has been considered as the "Spice Bowl of the World" since time immemorial. Consequently, all conquering tribes right from Assyrians and Babylonians, Arabians, Romans, Egyptians, to the British and the Portuguese, invaded India with one ambition—to benefit from the rich natural wealth, and Indian spices (Harrison, 2016).

Vedas, the most ancient Hindu scriptures, are considered as the earliest written documents mentioning about spices. For example, Rig Veda (around 1500–1200 Before Common Era, BCE) has references to different types of spices. Black pepper (*Piper nigrum*) has been mentioned in Yajur Veda (dating back to 1200–1000 BCE) as well (Harrison, 2016).

Utility for innumerable purposes could be the reason why allurement for spices can be traced back to the beginning of civilization. When there were no refrigerators, spices were used to retain the freshness of the cooked food for longer time, to do away with the unpleasant smell of decaying meat and to add taste and flavor to bland dishes. However, spices became an integral part of humans' everyday life, food, health and moods, as knowledge about their medicinal and other values unfolded (Narsimhan, 2009).

Black pepper, rightly known as the "King of Spices", is one such spice, which is the most important and most widely used across the world. Historically, black pepper has been held supreme among spices—courtesy, its characteristic pungency and flavor. Consequently, it has been indispensable in many food preparations, and it is the only spice that invariably gets served at your dining table! (Ravindran, 2000)

Chapter 1
PEPPER...THE BOTANIC HELEN OF TROY

Since antiquity, people from different civilizations have used black pepper for different purposes. For the ancient Indians it was a valuable drug, and now for most Indians it is a spice as well as a nutrient with various health benefits. For ancient Egyptians it was an essential ingredient for mummification (peppercorns were found stuffed in the nostrils of Ramesses II after his death in 1213 BCE). For civilized western people it is a spice, an essential additive to their food (Ravindran, 2000; Melissa, 2014).

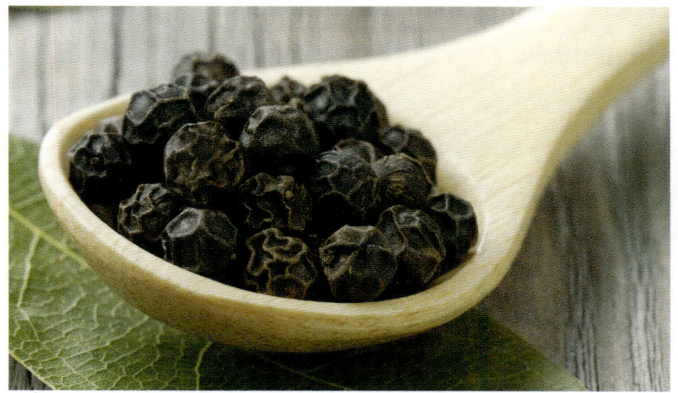
Dried black pepper fruits.

History of Black Pepper

The word "*pepper*" is derived from the Dravidian word for long pepper, 'pippali'. Ancient Greek and Latin turned pippali into the Latin *piper*, a term used by Romans to refer both black pepper and long pepper, as they believed that both of these spices were derived from the same plant. However, today's word "*pepper*" was derived from the old English word 'pipor' (Rawlinson, 2002).

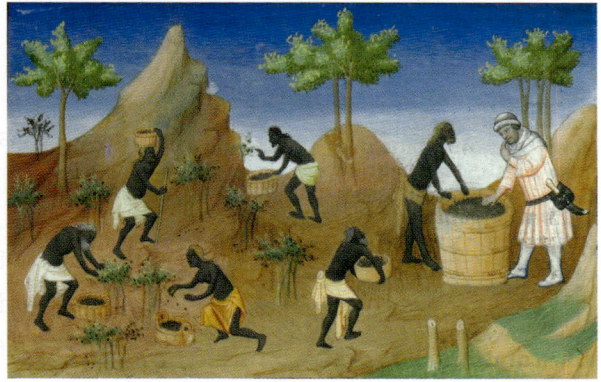
Black pepper harvesting in ancient India.
(Image source: schools-wikipedia.org)

The history of spices is certainly quite fascinating. The reason being, quest for this treasure has witnessed discovery of new lands, highs and lows of empires, flouting of trusts and favors, and rise and fall in the beliefs and practices of various religions.

Chapter 1
PEPPER...THE BOTANIC HELEN OF TROY

Though India has been the largest producer, consumer and exporter of black pepper since antiquity, during early days it was essentially a forest produce and people used to collect it from forests, where it was abundant. It was then traded with merchants in the local markets. Domestication of pepper appears to be a much later event (Ravindran, 2000).

Of all the spices, black pepper, particularly from Malabar Coast of India (also called Malabari peppercorns), has been historically the most significant. It made a good currency because of the flavor and thus intrinsic value, and was among the most valuable items of trade in ancient and medieval times (Narsimhan, 2009).

Plato, a famous Greek philosopher (429–347 BCE), described these tiny shrivelled berries as "small in quantity, great in virtue"—elucidating the covet for black pepper in European lands in earlier days, which became the symbol of power for the ruling class (Narsimhan, 2009).

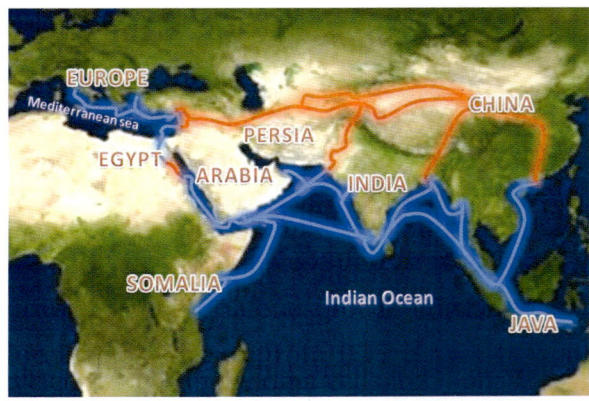

Ancient silk route (in red) and spice trade route (in blue).
(Image source: schools-wikipedia.org)

References to trading of black pepper between India and the West could be traced back to 3000–2000 BCE, when Assyrians and Babylonians were trading spices, including pepper, with the Malabar Coast of India. Well flourished Babylonian-China connection via Malabar Coast could be the reason that black pepper plants reached the far East and South-East Asian countries. In Eber's Papyrus (1550 BCE), there were references about pepper (Ravindran, 2000).

During the post-epic period of ancient Indian history—generally termed as 'the rationalistic period' (1500–600 BCE), Charaka, the famous physician, and Susruta, the ancient surgeon, mentioned about the medicinal uses of pepper. Panini, an ancient Sanskrit grammarian and a revered scholar, who also lived during this period, had written about the use of pepper for spicing wine (Ravindran, 2000).

Chapter 1
PEPPER...THE BOTANIC HELEN OF TROY

During 1000 BCE, Jews and the Arabs became the major traders by controlling spice trade and pepper routes, enjoying a huge monopoly of this lucrative business, which continued until the rise of the Roman Empire. Once the spice reached Mediterranean, it was Venice and Genoa—the Italian city-states, which held a monopoly on shipping lines. The Arabs, as middle men, safely guarded the secret of the country of origin and route to India from Egyptians and Greeks for a long time (Ravindran, 2000; Butler., 2013).

Romans controlled the pepper trade after conquest of Egypt in 40 Common Era (CE). Marcus Aurelius, the Roman emperor, was believed to tax all kinds of peppers, but black. However, when Alaric the Gothic conquered Rome (408 CE), he demanded a ransom of 3,000 pounds of pepper along with gold, silver, silk and hides (Ravindran, 2000; Toussaint-Samat, 2009).

Medicinal values of black pepper have been documented by Dioscorides, a Greek physician (40–90 CE), in his *Materia Medica*. The Greeks were so fond of pepper that it has been described as "Yavanapriya" (meaning beloved to the Greeks) in Sanskrit. The same has been corroborated by an ancient Tamil poet who had mentioned that "Yavanas (Greeks) use to bring in ships filled with gold and return loaded with pepper" (Ravindran, 2000).

Pepper found a place in majority of the recipes during 3rd century, as documented by Edward Gibbon in his book "The History of the Decline and Fall of the Roman Empire", stating that pepper was 'a favorite ingredient of the most expensive Roman cookery' (Nino, 2007).

The excellent trade relationships between China and the Malabar Coast reached its pinnacle during 1405–1433, as an estimated 50,000 catties (1 catty = 680 g) of pepper purchase was made by Chinese. As huge import of pepper into China triggered a fall in its price, during 5th century soldiers received pepper as part of their salary, albeit partially. In 1425, all government officials and private soldiers in China were given pepper as part of their salary (Ravindran, 2000).

At the beginning of the 14th century, lure for this prized spice attracted several sea farers, leading to many global explorations and circumnavigations of earth. This led to the beginning of the age of Christopher Columbus, Vasco da Gama, Sir Francis Drake and other voyagers. Though the main intention of Columbus was to obtain peppercorns and other exotic spices from India, he could not find Spice Islands on the west coast of India, instead, discovered America (Ravindran, 2000; Butler, 2013).

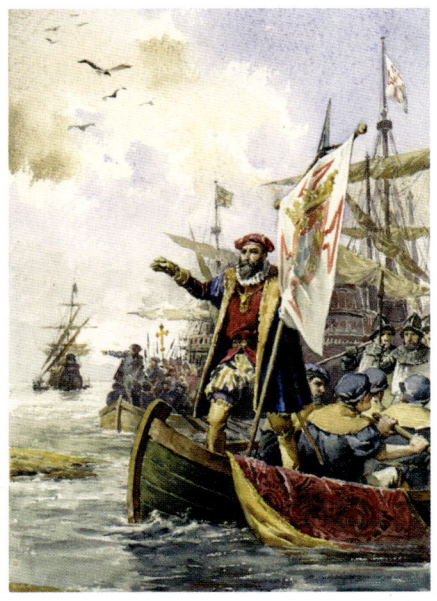

Arrival of Vasco da Gama at the Malabar Coast of India on May 20, 1498.
(Image source: www.newworldencyclopedia.org)

Authority of Portuguese Empire in the trade of black pepper began with the landing of Vasco da Gama, the Portuguese sailor, near Calicut on the Malabar Coast on May 20, 1498, which continued till 18th century. This indeed was also the beginning of the colonial era that ended the dominance of Arabs in Indian spices trade, permanently (Ravindran, 2000).

However, this Portugal monopoly was later broken by the English and Dutch. As the British Empire rose in prominence in the tropics, gradually it entered into trade agreements with all local rulers and took control of the spice trade by establishing British East India Company, a commercial establishment, supported by its dominant military (Ravindran, 2000; Melissa, 2014).

Eventually, the pepper plant, long grown in India, made its way to the New World. As a result, pepper was taken to countries like Indonesia, Malaysia, Vietnam, Brazil and others, which became major producers and exporters of pepper in the world market (Ravindran, 2000).

Black pepper, a highly valuable spice, influenced regional cuisines all over the world once its popularity quickly spread and became more easily and readily available. Common people were able to enjoy it, as the prices dropped. And people started introducing pepper into their diet along with their native spices and herbs. Ultimately, this led to the conception of typical spice blends, such as garam masala in India, ras el hanout in Morocco, quatre épices in France and Cajun and jerk blends in the Americas (Butler, 2013).

Chapter 1
PEPPER...THE BOTANIC HELEN OF TROY

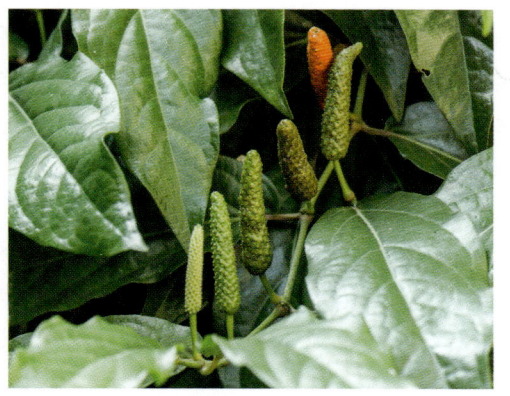

Long pepper (vine with berries/pepper corns).

Overall, till date, pepper continues to dominate the spice trade both in terms of volume and value, as well as the taste buds throughout the world. American Spice Trade Association (ASTA) has estimated that pepper accounted for about 20% of the total volume and value of world spices' trade in 2002 (Jaffee, 2005). Thus, pepper has become an indispensable part of cuisines around the world, as it subtly enlivening your foods, everyday!

Botanical Description

The genus *Piper* has more than 1,000 species, but the most well known species among them are black pepper (*Piper nigrum*), long pepper (*Piper longum*), kava kava (*Piper methysticum*) and betel (*Piper betle*). Black pepper originated in the tropical evergreen forests of the Western Ghats; and the Malabar Coast of India, became the center of trade from time immemorial. From here, pepper was taken throughout the tropical and sub-tropical regions of the world. Currently, around 26 countries are known to produce pepper (Ravindran, 2000; Ahmad et al., 2012).

Vernacular Names of Black Pepper

Sanskrit	*Maricha*
Hindi	*Golmirch, Kalimirch*
Malayalam	*Kurumulaku*
Kannada	*Karemensu*
Tamil	*Milagu, Kari*
Telugu	*Miriyalu, Maichamu*

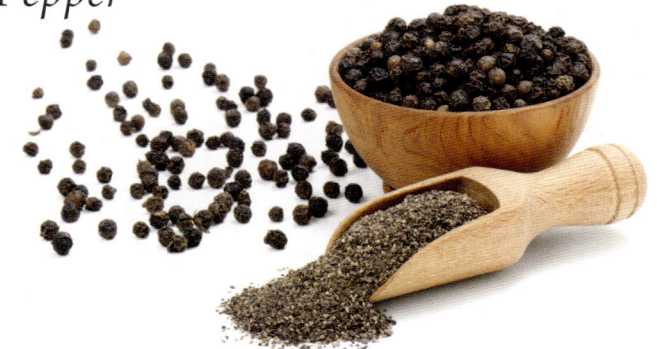

Chapter 1
PEPPER...THE BOTANIC HELEN OF TROY

Pepper plant is a perennial climber growing 4.5–7.5 m in height. It climbs with the aid of adventitious roots on trees or on artificial supports. The branches hang down forming a dense cylindrical canopy of foliage. Leaves are dark green, simple and alternate; broadly ovate in shape with acuminate apices, a thick texture and with 5–9 major veins.

The small sessile white flowers are borne in pendulous, dense, slender spikes of about 50 blossoms each. Berry-like fruits are globular or oblong, about 0.5–1 cm in diameter and contain a single seed. The fruit develops from an ovary with solitary, erect, basal, bitegmic, ovule. The fresh fruit is green and retains the pericarp (fruit wall). In the seed, the two integuments of the ovule are reduced to a dark layer between the fruit wall and the perisperm of the seed. However, the cellular traces of the two integuments are seen only in the micropylar region; so also the traces of the nuclear endosperm (Fig. 1A). The embryo is extremely minute.

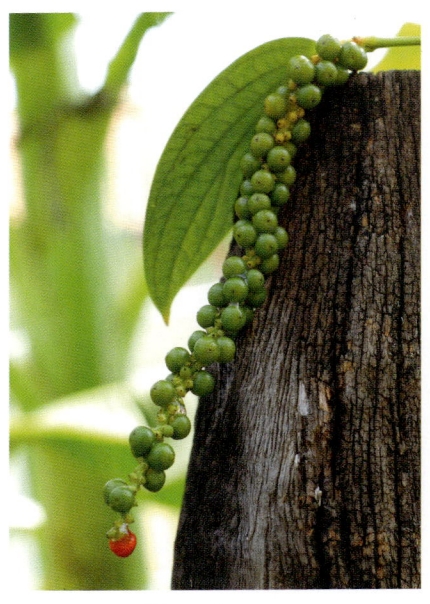

Piper nigrum
(vine with berries/pepper corns).

The green pericarp consists of 10–15 layers of cells. The epidermal cells and a few of hypodermal cells are converted into sclerified

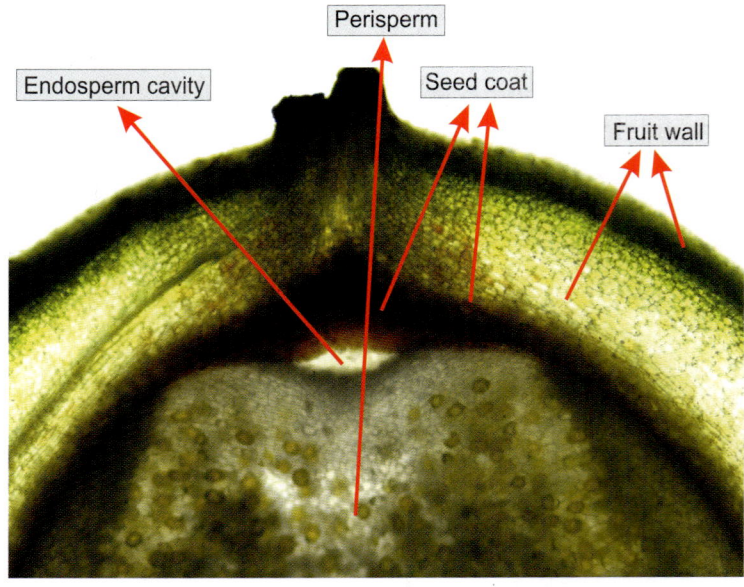

Fig. 1A: Longitudinal section of the micropylar region of a fresh green fruit (unstained).
(Image source: Sami Labs)

cells, while the most inner part of the pericarp has a distinct inner epidermal layer, adjacent to which are a number of oil cavities. The intervening layers are parenchymatous and filled with chloroplasts, which fluoresce to a red color under fluorescence microscope. A number of vascular bundles are found in this zone (Fig. 1B and 1C). The whole pericarp dries up, loses its cellular nature and becomes black in the mature condition. The black fruits contain mainly remnants of the seed coat in the form of a black amorphous surface layer and the perisperm as well as surface grooves, which are responsible for its uneven nature.

The major part of the seed is perisperm, which represents nucellus of the ovule. The perisperm cells are essentially parenchymatous and contain oils, oleoresins, starch grains and alkaloids.

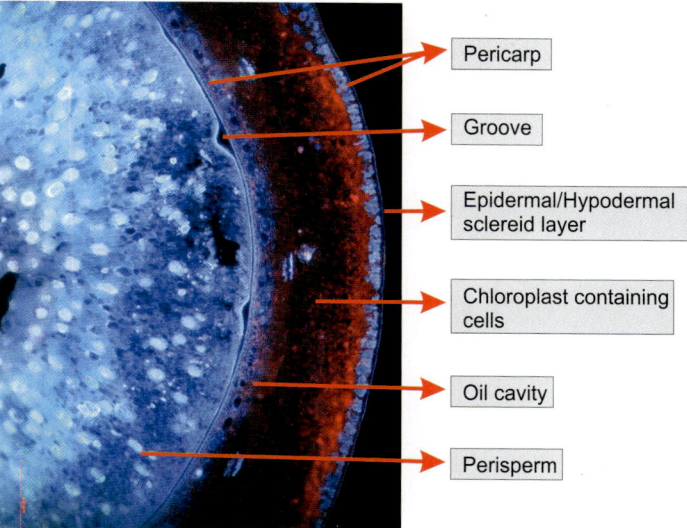

Fig. 1B: A portion of transverse section of fresh green fruit - viewed under fluorescence microscope (UV illumination).
(Image source: Sami Labs)

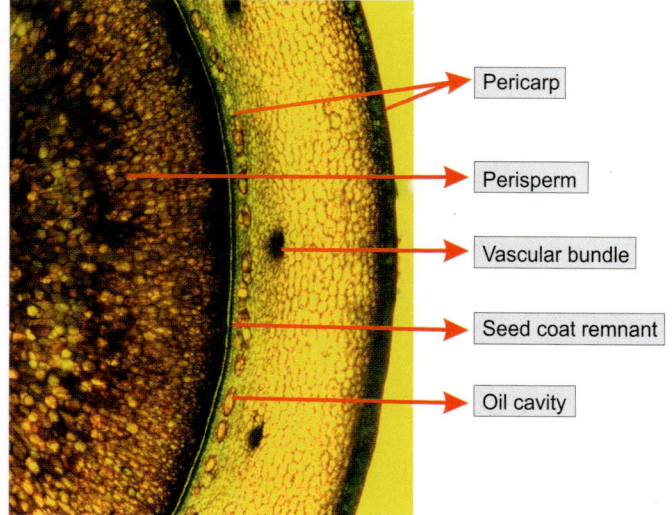

Fig. 1C: A portion of transverse section of fresh green fruit stained with Toluidine Blue O - viewed under blue filters.
(Image source: Sami Labs)

Chemistry

Apart from very well known physiological properties and effective management of various health conditions, black pepper is also acknowledged for its intrinsic quality—*the spiciness*—characterized by its distinct sharp and pungent qualities.

Piperine, the alkaloid found both in the fresh green fruit and in the seed of black pepper, is the major component and the most recognized compound that contributes to its pungency, whereas essential oil constituents like α- and β-pinene, limonene, myrcene, linalool, α-phellandrene, sabinene, β-caryophyllene, germacrene-D impart the characteristic aroma and flavor (Sruthi et al., 2013). Piperine is present in the highest concentration of all secondary compounds in the plant seed (Scott et al., 2008).

In 1820, Hans Christian Ørstedt, a Dutch chemist, first isolated piperine, the bioactive and pungent component from the fruits of *Piper nigrum* (Srinivasan, 2009). Bordner and Mullins were the first to publish single crystal diffractometry of piperine in 1974 (Bordner and Mullins, 1974). Murthy and Bhattacharya have reported that volatile oil present in the cells of pericarp is responsible for the characteristic odor of black pepper (Murthy and Bhattacharya, 2008).

At least three polymorphs of piperine belonging to monoclinic crystal system are known. The optical microscopy images of these three polymorphs are shown in Fig. 1D.

Form II and III are monotropically related to form I. Form II and III have enhanced solubility in water relative to form I. Form I is thermodynamically the most stable form (Pfund et al., 2015).

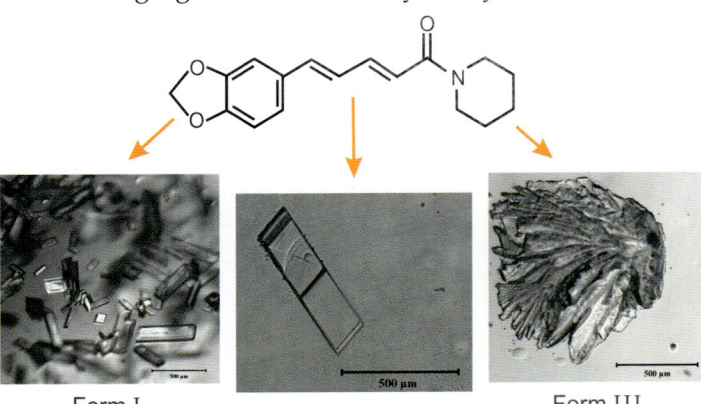

Fig. 1D: Optical microscopy of piperine forms I, II and III.
(Reproduced from Pfund et al., 2015)

Chapter 1
PEPPER...THE BOTANIC HELEN OF TROY

Black Pepper, an Age-old Medicine

Black pepper has been used not only in human diets but also in various traditional medicines and home remedies since ages. In India, black pepper figures in remedies in Ayurveda and other alternative traditional systems of medicine, viz. Siddha and Unani.

Black pepper is specifically cited in Ayurveda for internal treatments (e.g. fevers, gastric and abdominal disorders, and urinary problems) as well as for external treatments (e.g. rheumatism, neuralgia, boils etc.). Black pepper has also been known to treat respiratory diseases (e.g. asthma, bronchitis), dysentery, pyrexia and insomnia, as a part of Indian folk medicine (Srinivasan, 2009). However, it appears that its extensive generalized use was to enhance the effects of many herbal remedies. Ayurvedic physicians have been prescribing black pepper for hundreds of years, a practice which may have enhanced the pharmacological actions of other compounds in traditional herbal medicines.

Additionally, black pepper is a vital ingredient of many remedies in the traditional Ayurvedic system of medicine in India. For example, black pepper is a component of "trikatu" (meaning three acrids) along with long pepper (*Piper longum*) and ginger (*Zingiber officinale*) in equal proportions. According to ancient Ayurvedic *Materia Medica*

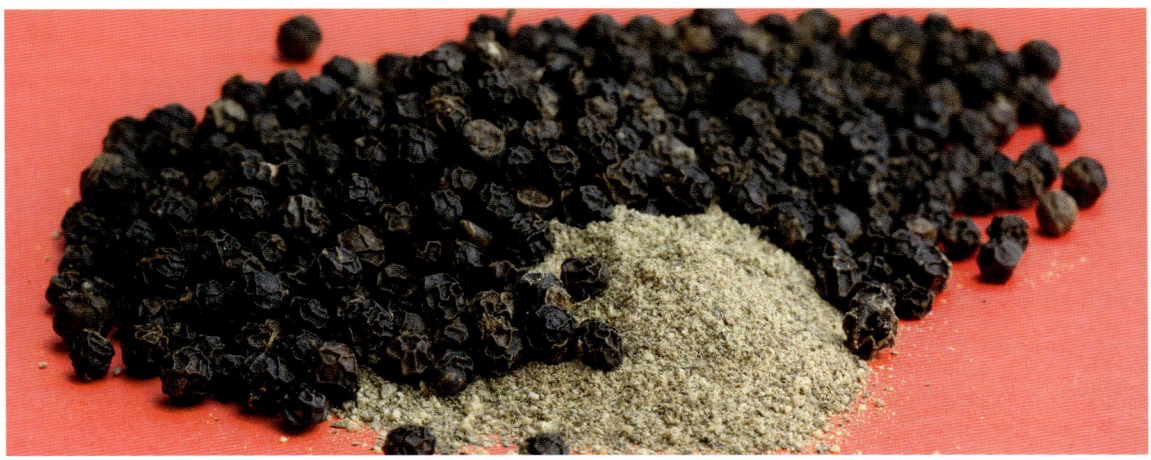
Dried black pepper corns and its crushed powder.

(600–300 BCE), trikatu is widely used in combination with other Ayurvedic medications for a range of health conditions (Srinivasan, 2009).

Out of 370 compound formulations listed in Handbook of Domestic Medicines and Common Ayurvedic Remedies, 210 contain either trikatu or its individual ingredients (Johri and Zutshi, 1992).

There are hardly any Ayurvedic prescriptions that are free from these three acrids. It is believed that trikatu aims to correct the imbalance of the three "doshas" (meaning psychophysical components of the human body) that can lead to different disease conditions (Srinivasan, 2009).

Hence, one could realize that wide-ranging use of black pepper in India is unprecedented in other medical systems and areas of the rest of the world.

Genetic Diversity of Piper nigrum

The genus *Piper* includes the most valuable and economically important spice crop, black pepper. Although this crop has become a synonym for the Asian continent, particularly the Western Ghats of Indian peninsula, countries like Malaysia, Indonesia, Thailand, Vietnam, China and Sri Lanka, as well as South American countries like Brazil and Madagascar are also known for the cultivation of black pepper.

As per cytological studies the basic chromosome number of *Piper* species is $x = 13$, whereas *Piper nigrum* is tetraploid ($2n = 52$). Cross-pollination between different species of *Piper* when more than one species climbed up the same support trees is thought to be one of the evolutionary parameters for polyploidy in *Piper nigrum*. However, subsequent gene flow might have been restricted in these progenies due to the absence of pollen transfer mechanism, while successful vegetative propagation ensured survival as well as spread of these species (Joy et al., 2007).

To date, more than 100 cultivars of black pepper have been known. It is believed that initially cultivars from the wild might have been domesticated and selected (Ravindran, 2000).

However, in the current day scenario, diversity among *Piper nigrum* cultivars, which are vegetatively propagated by farmers through cuttings, depends on breeding and conservation programs based on good fruit set, pungency etc. Additionally, several other factors, such as change in tropical climates, development of diseases, use of pesticides influence the quality and production (i.e. crop loss) of black pepper. As a result, despite being a crop with agricultural and economic importance, knowledge of black pepper genetics is presently very limited (Gordo et al., 2012).

Characterization and quantification of genetic diversity among the available germplasm is imperative for crop improvement programs. In recent years, techniques like amplified fragments length polymorphism, novel polymerase chain reaction (PCR) based assays and next-generation sequencing like ribonucleic acid (RNA) Seq technology have offered immense opportunity for the fast access to genetic information, deoxyribonucleic acid (DNA) polymorphism and transcriptomes of black pepper (Joy et al., 2007; Gordo et al., 2012).

Chapter 2

Mechanism of Bioenhancement by Piperine

Although advancements in modern pharmaceutical research has led to the introduction of new molecules with novel mechanism of action, several promising molecules have encountered the issue of poor bioavailability, particularly upon oral ingestion.

Bioavailability refers to the rate and extent to which a therapeutically active substance enters the circulation and reaches the target site(s) to exert its biological action(s). The concern related to bioavailability is due to various causes, such as poor permeation across the gastrointestinal epithelial cells because of meagre membrane permeability (probably due to their low lipophilicity and zwitterionic character at physiological pH) or because of poor water solubility or efflux by P-glycoprotein (P-gp), an adenosine triphosphate (ATP) dependent drug efflux pump (Kang *et al.*, 2009).

Thus, it becomes imperative to improve the oral absorption and bioavailability of nutrients/drugs. As a result, numerous approaches have been adopted to overcome such bioavailability-related issues. Some of the approaches include: use of absorption enhancers, pronutrients/prodrugs and application of P-gp inhibitors (Kang *et al.*, 2009).

Chapter 2
MECHANISM OF BIOENHANCEMENT BY PIPERINE

Ayurveda has been playing a major role in the drug discovery process. In recent years, there has been growing interest on using natural compounds to enhance the bioavailability of nutrients/drugs, which has guided a radical change in the process of drug delivery (Atal and Bedi, 2010).

Piperine, a Natural Bioenhancer

Bioenhancer is an agent capable of enhancing bioavailability and bioefficiency of a particular drug/nutrient with which it is combined. In the case of piperine the term *"bioavailability enhancer"* was first coined by Indian scientists from Indian Institute of Integrative Medicine (IIIM), Jammu (formerly known as Regional Research Laboratory; RRL), where drug bioavailability enhancement property of piperine was first discovered and scientifically validated in 1979 (Atal and Bedi, 2010).

Various mechanisms have been attributed to the bioavailability enhancing activity of natural compounds from medicinal plants, including increased blood supply to the gastrointestinal tract, increase in intestinal brush border membrane fluidity, decreased hydrochloric acid secretion thus preventing breakdown of some drugs, inhibition of enzymes involved in drug metabolism and inhibition of ATP-dependent drug efflux proteins.

Upon scrutinizing a list of formulations used for numerous disease conditions, it was found that either 'trikatu' or one of its three ingredients has a key role to play in enhancing drug/nutrient bioavailability when given orally. Hence, it has now been considered that some of the compounds of natural origin improve the absorption and bioavailability of co-administered nutrients and drugs, which is relatively very straightforward and safe (Kang *et al.*, 2009; Atal and Bedi, 2010).

Mechanism of Action of Piperine

Prescription medicines as well as herbal constituents undergo a series of events involving biotransformation with varied absorption profiles. Thus, consumption of natural products—known to improve bioavailability and absorption resulting in enhanced efficacy, is gaining importance around the world.

One such natural product that has been most widely used in human diet for a long time is black pepper or its major active component, piperine. Several reports have documented bioenhancement of a number of therapeutic and/or nutritional agents as well as other phytochemicals by piperine (Srinivasan, 2007; Han, 2011).

The mechanism by which piperine enhances the drug bioavailability may be explained by following possible explanations:

- Modulation of P-glycoprotein-mediated drug/nutrient efflux
- Modulation of metabolic enzymes involved in biotransformation of drugs/nutrients
- Enhanced intestinal absorption
- Thermogenesis

Modulation of P-glycoprotein-mediated Drug/Nutrient Efflux

In recent times, understanding of food-mediated changes in cellular function, especially, in the expression and function of membrane transporter proteins has preceded the growing popularity of herbs and spices, such as black pepper, as complementary medicines. As a result, their impact on the therapeutic outcome has been very much evident. One such transporter that has been widely investigated is the P-gp efflux pump.

P-glycoprotein, a member of the superfamily of ATP-binding cassette of transporters, is the product of the multidrug resistance gene, MDR1 (ABCB1), in humans. It was first characterized as an ATP-dependent transporter—a transmembrane protein consisting of 1,280 amino acids (molecular mass ~170 kDa), responsible for the efflux of chemotherapeutic agents in drug-resistant cancer cells. Since then, it has been known to have wide tissue distribution and substrate specificity. As a result, P-gp efflux activity has been implicated as the underlying mechanism of a wide range of drug-drug and drug-food interactions that are of clinical significance (Han *et al.*, 2008; Zhang *et al.*, 2009; Han, 2011).

Functional P-gp is also expressed in normal epithelial cells, such as the canalicular surface of hepatocytes, the apical membrane of proximal renal tubular cells and the brush border membrane of intestinal enterocytes. Due to its ubiquitous distribution throughout the body tissues, P-gp is believed to exhibit defensive roles; for example, P-gp in the intestine is thought to limit the absorption of environmental and dietary toxins, whereas P-gp in the liver and kidney aids elimination of toxins through biliary and urinary excretion, respectively.

Structurally, P-gp molecule has as many as four substrate-binding sites, each with a different binding specificity—which enables it to simultaneously bind with different substrates and transport a wide range of structurally unrelated compounds out of cells. P-glycoprotein can potentially decrease the absorption, oral bioavailability as well as retention time of a number

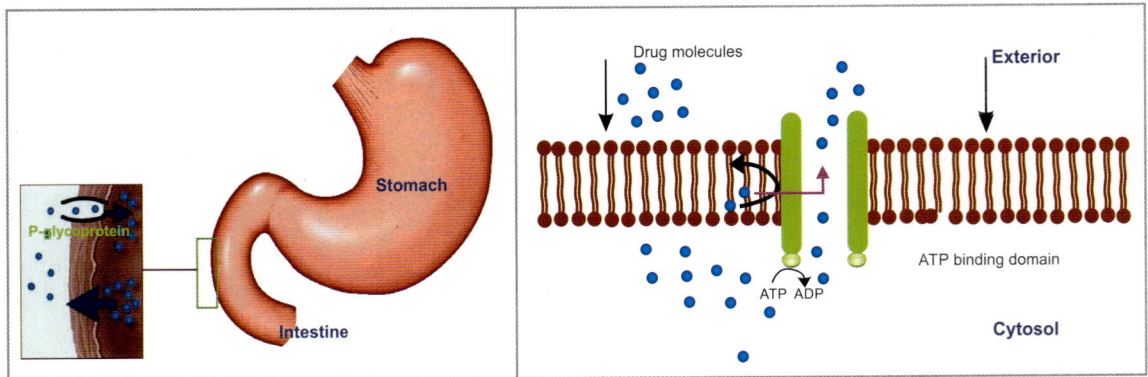

Fig. 2A: P-glycoprotein-mediated xenobiotic efflux pump. (Reproduced from Amin, 2013)
Several drugs/nutrients, which are structurally diverse in nature, get extruded by P-gp out of the cells. This ATP-dependent transporter is also responsible for substantial extrusion of a number of substrates (even weak or less permeable), usually hydrophobic ones. Thus, P-gp can potentially decrease the retention time of xenobiotics, and in turn their absorption and oral bioavailability.

of drugs/nutrients (Fig. 2A). Hence, efflux mechanism mediated through P-gp influencing xenobiotic permeability across cell membrane is believed to modulate various functional activities, including cancer chemotherapy, drug-drug and drug-food interactions as well as oral drug/nutrient bioavailability. Thus, agents that have the ability to influence the functional activity or cellular expression of P-gp (i.e. by inhibiting competitively or non-competitively) could alter the intestinal absorption or the renal and biliary excretion of various P-gp substrates—lead to the clinically important pharmacokinetic or pharmacodynamic modifications (Fig. 2B) (Zhou et al., 2004; Han et al., 2008; Zhang et al., 2009; Han, 2011; Amin, 2013).

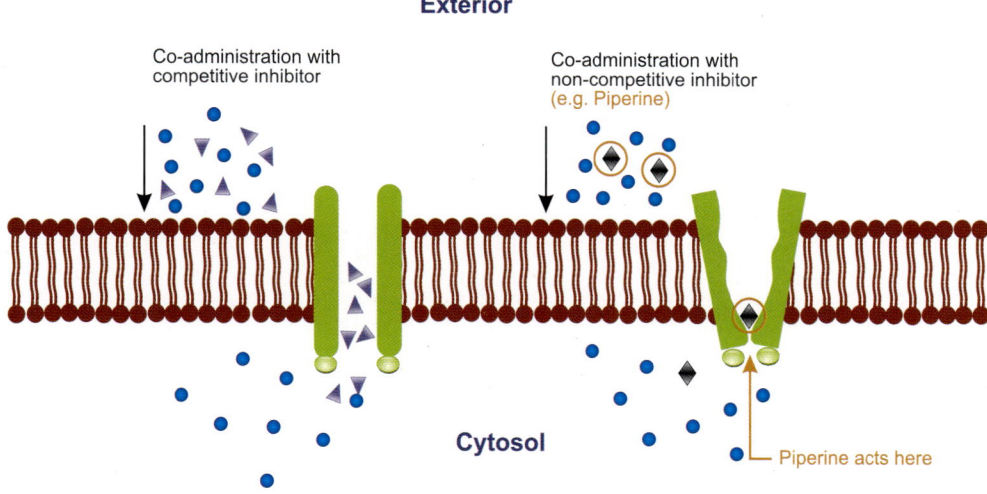

Fig. 2B: Prevention of drug/nutrient efflux by inhibiting of P-glycoprotein. (Reproduced from Amin, 2013)
Several agents are believed to inhibit P-gp-mediated efflux pump (competitively or non-competitively) and thus help enhance oral drug/nutrient bioavailability and absorption. For example, piperine is considered to act non-competitively on the P-gp-dependent efflux pump.

Of late, much of the research on P-gp-mediated efflux mechanism at molecular and biochemical levels has focused on the effect of co-administration of P-gp inhibitors, such as dietary phytochemicals, piperine, for example, on the absorption, distribution and elimination of xenobiotics, including drugs.

Clinical significance of concurrent use of piperine on the efficiency of co-administered drugs/nutrients has been investigated by several researchers. Furthermore, a vast amount of data has been published in the recent past supporting modulation of functional activity or gene expression of P-gp by piperine (Zhou et al., 2004; Han et al., 2008; Zhang et al., 2009; Han, 2011; Amin, 2013).

Similar observations were made by Han et al. when co-administered piperine (50–100 µM) abolished the polarity of digoxin transport in Caco-2 and L-MDR1 cell monolayers, which was comparable to the effect of 100 µM of verapamil, a calcium channel blocker and a potent P-gp inhibitor. However, piperine elevated the P-gp protein activity and expression in Caco-2 cell cultures following prolonged co-exposure for 48 h or 72 h, which was also emulated as elevated intestinal P-gp expression following intragastric administration of piperine for 14 days although hepatic P-gp was downregulated, while the renal P-gp level remained unaffected.

The explanation for such finding was that piperine-mediated P-gp induction could be occurring at the transcriptional level rather than during cell differentiation, which may not always give rise to functional protein. Additionally, considering that the Caco-2 cells are a Pregnane X Receptor (PXR) deficient cell line, piperine might have modulated the P-gp expression through a mechanism that is different from established P-gp modulators, such as rifampicin and St John's wort, which regulate the cellular expression of P-gp by a PXR-dependent mechanism. Furthermore, the reversibility of the piperine-mediated P-gp induction effect, as demonstrated in the Caco-2 cell monolayers, could also signify that time-dependent decline of tissue P-gp to baseline levels would reduce the impact of dietary piperine on pharmacokinetics of nutrients, thus making piperine a relatively safer bioenhancer with no associated drug interactions in the clinic (Han et al., 2008).

Overall, several study reports strongly advocate that piperine could be an effective bioenhancer owing to its influence on P-gp-mediated drugs/nutrients efflux mechanism.

Modulation of Metabolic Enzymes involved in Biotransformation of Drugs/Nutrients

Metabolism is a general term used to describe chemical transformation of xenobiotics and endogenous nutrients, such as proteins, carbohydrates and fats, within or outside the body. It is an essential biological process or rather pharmacokinetic process, which restricts the life of a substance in the body by converting lipid-soluble and non-polar substances into more water-soluble and polar ones—thus, eliminating them out of the body by various processes.

Biotransformation is a specific term used to describe chemical transformation of xenobiotics in the body or living organism. A number of enzymes are involved in the biotransformation of xenobiotics, including drugs and nutrients, and are divided into phase I and phase II enzymes, depending upon the phase of the biotransformation they are involved in (Jancova et al., 2010).

Glucuronidation is a phase II biotransformation reaction, wherein addition of glucuronic acid to a substrate is often involved in transforming respective conjugates more hydrophilic.

Hence, interaction of piperine with enzymes that participate in drug metabolism has been attributed as one of the reasons for its bioenhancing effect. It has also been noted that piperine interacts with the process of oxidative phosphorylation or the process of activation/deactivation of certain metabolic pathways, thus slowing down the metabolism and biodegradation of drugs—resulting in improved plasma levels of drugs—more available for pharmacological action (Wadhwa et al., 2014).

To understand the interaction of piperine with enzymes involved in drug biotransformation, hepatic tissues were studied *in vitro* and *in vivo*. Piperine exhibited a dose-dependent inhibition of arylhydrocarbon hydroxylation, ethylmorphine-N-demethylation, 7-ethoxycoumarin-O-deethylation and 3-hydroxy-benzo(a)pyrene (3-OH-BAP) glucuronidation in rat liver postmitochondrial supernatant *in vitro*.

Similarly, oral administration of piperine in rats significantly inhibited the hepatic arylhydrocarbon hydroxylase and Uridine 5'-diphospho-glucuronosyltransferase (UDP-glucuronosyltransferase, UGT) activities. In addition, oral and intraperitoneal administration of piperine also enhanced hexobarbital-induced sleeping time as well as zoxazolamine paralysis time in mice at half the dose of SKF-525A, a reference compound. Overall, authors concluded that piperine could be a potent inhibitor of drug metabolism (Atal *et al.*, 1985).

The basis of inhibition of glucuronidation by piperine (Fig. 3) was further investigated by Singh *et al.* in intact epithelial cells isolated from small intestine of guinea pig. Here, rate of glucuronidation of 3-OH-BAP and UDP-glucuronic acid (UDPGA) content was evaluated. The glucuronidation of 3-OH-BAP was dependent on the duration of incubation, cellular protein and endogenous UDPGA concentration. Piperine was found to decrease the cellular content of UDPGA and the rate of glucuronidation. Piperine also produced a non-competitive inhibition of hepatic microsomal UGT with inhibitory constant (K_i) of 70 μM (Singh *et al.*, 1986).

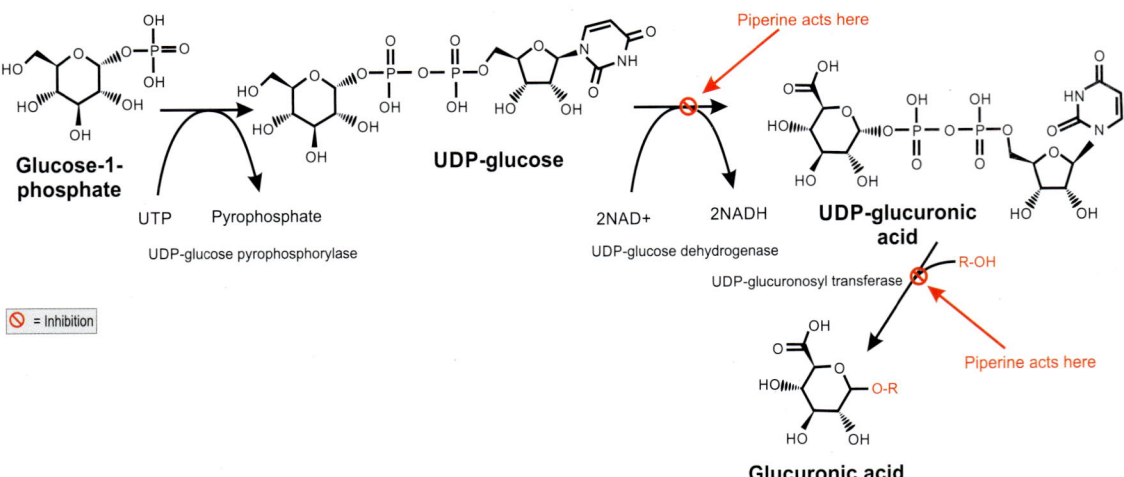

Fig. 3: Action of glucuronidation inhibition by piperine.

Piperine is thought to be inhibiting glucuronidation, a process by which human body eliminates various xenobiotics from the body, by inhibiting enzymes like UDP-glucose dehydrogenase and UDP-glucuronosyl transferase, and in turn lowering the levels of endogenous glucuronic acid.

Another study from Reen *et al.* examined the effects of piperine on UDP-glucose dehydrogenase (UDP-GDH) and glucuronidation potentials in liver and intestine of rat and guinea pig. Results proved that piperine produced a concentration-dependent, reversible, strong, non-competitive and equipotent inhibition of UDP-GDH in both tissues. However, piperine reduced the UDPGA contents in enterocytes of guinea pig small intestine more significantly than in rat hepatocytes. In addition, piperine showed varied UGT inhibitory activity in liver and intestine of rat. Piperine showed weak inhibition of UGT1A1 activity, but it did not influence UGT2B1 activity in the liver. In contrast, in a guinea pig small intestine, piperine showed significant inhibition of both these activities at a much lower concentration.

Taken together, the results inferred that piperine is a potent inhibitor of UDP-GDH—by virtue of conjugated double bonds of the molecule, and it exerts stronger effects on intestinal glucuronidation than in the rat liver. This could be due to the fact that small intestine is very rich in glucuronidation potential and several drugs/nutrients (having phenolic hydroxyl groups as the pharmacologically active substituents) are possibly attractive substrates for glucuronidation during intestinal extraction. Therefore, piperine might be a helpful agent against intestinal conjugation of such agents (Reen et al., 1993).

Enhanced Intestinal Absorption

For a drug/nutrient to be transported from lumen of the gut into the systemic circulation, it must pass through the epithelial barrier of intestinal mucosa. Several anatomical and biological barriers limit the rate of penetration of drugs/nutrients into the epithelial membrane, particularly when given orally. Intestinal epithelium is one such barrier, with many complex structures, that restricts the transfer of drugs/nutrients from the gastrointestinal tract to the systemic circulation. Numerous absorption pathways play a major role in assisting transportation of drugs/nutrients that are less permeable (Fig. 4).

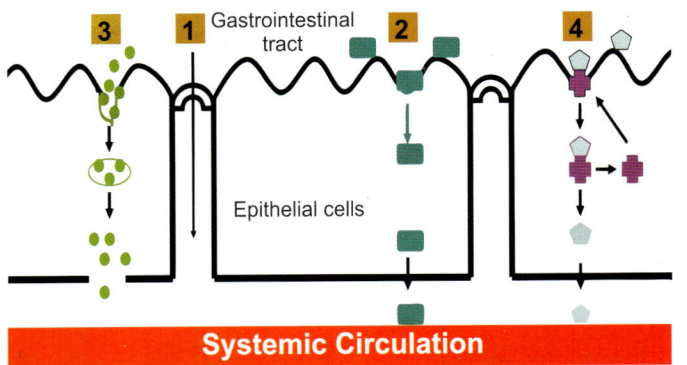

Fig. 4: Various intestinal absorption pathways.
(Reproduced from Kang *et al.*, 2009)

1. Paracellular and transcellular transport system 2. Transcellular passive diffusion 3. Transcellular endocytosis
4. Carrier-mediated transport system

Epithelial barrier of the intestinal mucosa influences absorption and therapeutic effect of large number of xenobiotics, particularly upon oral ingestion. Several barriers regulate entry of xenobiotics into systemic circulation.

Therefore, compounds that help to overcome such membrane dynamics and permeation characteristics would be of great utility in enhancing the absorption of drugs/nutrients which are poorly bioavailable upon oral ingestion.

The mechanism of bioenhancing property of piperine can thus be explained, at least in part, by improved absorption resulting from modulation of cell membrane fluidity. With this hypothesis, Khajuria *et al.* performed a membrane fluidity test using an apolar fluorescent probe, pyrene (which measures the fluid properties of hydrocarbon core). Results showed increased intestinal brush border membrane fluidity. It was also observed that activities of leucine aminopeptidase and glycylglycine dipeptidase were enhanced, which could be attributed to the alteration in enzyme kinetics by piperine. It was suggested that due to its apolar nature, piperine could modulate the membrane dynamics by interacting with surrounding lipids and hydrophobic portions in the protein vicinity, which may decrease the tendency of membrane lipids to act as stearic constrains to enzyme proteins, and thus modify enzyme conformation.

Additional ultra structural studies demonstrated an increase in microvilli length in the presence of piperine—suggesting that piperine might induce alterations in membrane dynamics and permeation characteristics, resulting in an enlarged absorptive surface of small intestine—thus, assisting efficient permeation through the epithelial barrier (Khajuria *et al.*, 2002).

Corroborating results were reported by Prakash and Srinivasan when they studied beneficial effect of piperine (0.02%) and black pepper (0.5%) for 8 weeks in experimental rats on:

i) the membrane fluidity of intestinal brush border membrane

ii) the activity of intestinal membrane-bound enzymes

iii) ultrastructural alterations in the intestinal epithelium

An increased brush border membrane fluidity was observed, which was further corroborated with a decreased cholesterol:phospholipid ratio in the jejunal and ileal regions of the intestine. Treatment groups showed stimulated activities of brush border membrane enzymes (glycylglycine dipeptidase, leucine aminopeptidase and γ-glutamyl transpeptidase) in the jejunal mucosa—suggesting the possible modulating effect of piperine on the membrane dynamics, as discussed above.

Furthermore, scanning electronic microscopy of the intestinal villi revealed alterations in the ultrastructure, especially an increase in microvilli length and perimeter—a favorable increase in the absorptive surface of the small intestine—thus, increasing bioavailability of micronutrients (Prakash and Srinivasan, 2010).

Overall, it was evident that piperine exhibited bioenhancing quality by modifying brush border membrane fluidity and passive permeability property, associated with increased absorptive surface of the small intestine.

The bioavailability of nutritional supplements is dependent on absorption, one of the physiological functions of the digestive tract. As a result, several elaborate systems of molecular sensors have been found to regulate the motor and secretory activity of the gastrointestinal tract. Transient receptor potential (TRP) channels, non-selective cation channels are the prominent among these molecular sensors, whose distinct chemical and physical modalities are specific to digestive system (Holzer, 2011a).

Vanniloid receptor-1, the first member of the vanilloid (V) subgroup of TRP channels and is a capsaicin receptor, which is now referred to as TRPV1. Vanilloid receptors like TRPV1, embedded on the surface of nerve cells that are ubiquitously distributed within the muscle layer, blood vessels and mucosa of the gastrointestinal tract are believed to influence piperine-mediated enhanced intestinal absorption.

Piperine is thought to improve the absorption of nutritional supplements by binding to the vanilloid receptor by triggering the activation of the membrane-bound enzyme, adenylyl cyclase. This enzyme further catalyzes the synthesis of cyclic adenosine monophosphate (cAMP), a derivative of ATP and a "second messenger", important in many biological processes. This further results in cAMP-activated protein kinase A (PKA), which is involved in modulating various physiological responses depending on the cell type, e.g. PKA inhibits intestinal motility and dilates blood vessels of the gastrointestinal tract (Geppetti and Trevisani, 2004; Rosenbaum and Simon, 2007; Holzer, 2011b).

Hence, these physiological changes are deemed to enhance digestion, better absorption and temperature rise in the gut.

Influence of spices on taste and digestive properties, which are the resultant of neuronal and vascular effects, are very well known. However, effect of direct interaction of spices with gastrointestinal epithelia was little known until Jensen-Jarolim *et al.* studied the influence of some selected spices and their major components.

An intestinal epithelial cell line (HCT-8), derived from a human ileocecal adenocarcinoma, was used to evaluate the effects of black pepper and piperine on transepithelial electrical resistance, a quantitative technique to measure the integrity of tight junction dynamics of endothelial and epithelial monolayers, permeability and morphological alterations of tight junctions.

Results suggested contrasting effects on the permeability of intestinal epithelia, with chilli pepper and capsaicin showing significantly decreased transepithelial electrical resistance and increase in permeability, while black pepper and piperine significantly increased transepithelial electrical resistance and lowered the permeability (Jensen-Jarolim et al., 1998).

Based on the study outcome and other reports (Takeuchi et al., 1994) suggesting possible relationship between increased gastrointestinal permeability and pathogenesis of certain gastrointestinal diseases, it could be ascertained that theoretically piperine is devoid of causing deleterious effects on the digestive system, unlike capsaicin, by maintaining low permeability and high transepithelial electrical resistance. Additionally, piperine helps in maintaining gastrointestinal well being by virtue of enhanced nutrient absorption, which is a physiological process, as against pathologically increased gastrointestinal permeability witnessed with capsaicin.

Piperine has also been postulated to display its bioenhancing action via several other mechanisms that advance intestinal drug absorption, viz. reduction in hydrochloric acid secretion and increase in gastrointestinal blood supply, inhibition of gastrointestinal transit (GT), gastric emptying (GE) time and intestinal motility, and cholagogous effect (Kesarwani et al, 2013).

Thermogenesis

One of the major sources of concern as regards to the poor nutritional status of any subject population is the conflict between poor nutrient bioavailability and better health, and nutritional effectiveness. Therefore, the principle is that one can consume highly nutritious food but the body will be benefitted only if it can absorb the nutrients from it.

It is well known that spices and herbs are used to give flavor to foods and drinks since primeval time without adding calories, hence consumption of spiced foods or herbal drinks are thought to be good for burning calories and in some cases to induce satiety. Therefore, it is suggested that these ingredients can realistically be considered as functional agents that could help in preventing a positive energy balance and improved nutrient absorption (Westerterp-Plantenga et al, 2006).

Chapter 2
MECHANISM OF BIOENHANCEMENT BY PIPERINE

The quote *"It is quite surprising that the use of pepper has come so much in fashion, its only desirable quality being certain pungency; and yet it is for this that we import it all the way from India!"*, attributed to Pliny the Elder, a Roman author, naturalist and natural philosopher, sums it all about widespread popularity of black pepper across the world, since prehistoric times (Ravindran, 2000).

The 'hot' or spicy taste of black pepper is no accident but a manifestation of the biological activity of some of the phytochemicals present in it, most notably, piperine. Consequently, it has now been realized scientifically that the 'pungency' of piperine is accompanied by a chain of biochemical and physiological reactions — resulting in generating a warmth or heat sensation in the body. This 'natural feeling' induced by piperine may have a broader influence on the body than just a pleasant sensory perception.

In general, this phenomenon of 'warmth feeling' could well be explained as a signal from the body that the digestion process followed by absorption is underway, once food is consumed. We won't feel that warmth when the digestion and absorption processes are not in order. In other words, our food is not fuelling us with enough life-supporting nutrients for the body's metabolic process, and in turn the metabolic process does not respond by generating the heat energy signal. This thermic effect of nutrients from food that empowers the process of energy production as a result of food metabolism in the body is termed as *'dietary thermogenesis'* or *'food-induced thermogenesis'* (Majeed et al, 1999).

Recently, a section of nutrition science started witnessing advanced discoveries. Consequently, inter-relation between food and functional food supplements has gained the importance around the concept of thermogenesis and nutrition absorption. While food is a principal cause of thermogenesis, the pungent principles, such as piperine are hypothesized to mimic and even support the process of food-induced thermogenesis.

Piperine, a Natural Thermonutrient

Another possible mechanism which underlines the activity of piperine as a bioenhancer in nutrient absorption is based on its ability to generate thermogenesis. According to Micevych *et al.*, the proposed mechanism highlighting inhibition of pain stimulus transmission followed by desensitization of pain receptors (also called as thermoreceptors) by piperine (both locally, at nerve endings as well as systemically, throughout the nervous system) might spell out its thermogenic action (Micevych *et al.*, 1983).

The leading theory that speaks about food-induced thermogenesis involves autonomous nervous system (ANS), which is known to regulate both sides of the energy balance equation and is an important regulator of energy expenditure. Thus, possible connection of ANS with thermogenesis is suggested by the ability of epinephrine and norepinephrine, the ANS hormones, to control biochemical mechanisms that lead either to an increased use of ATP, a coenzyme for intracellular energy transfer or enhanced heat generation as a result of increased rate of mitochondrial oxidation with poor coupling of ATP synthesis. Several studies have demonstrated enhanced thermogenesis in response to the infusion of norepinephrine or epinephrine (Westerterp-Plantenga *et al.*, 2006). It has also been found that epinephrine increases levels of cAMP, which in turn triggers production of heat energy, for example, by activating a host of enzymes, contraction of muscles (Majeed *et al.*, 1999).

Hence, when transformation of chemical energy into heat energy or thermogenesis is completed, demand for new nutrients rises to sustain the process. Accordingly, food-induced thermogenesis can be seen as a mechanism by which the intestinal absorption is facilitated.

Black pepper has also been understood to elevate the levels of circulating thyroid hormones—the basic participants in thermogenesis. As a result, both adrenergic and thyroid hormones work together to mediate a sustained thermogenic effect. Although the effect mediated by epinephrine and norepinephrine is transient, thyroid hormones are known to provide long-lasting response, thus, they take over and regulate the thermogenesis for longer duration (Majeed et al., 1999).

The stimulatory effect of pungent principles, such as piperine has also been attributed to the involvement of a TRPV1-linked thermogenic mechanism. This receptor is likely the key mediator of the effects of piperine on metabolism (Westerterp-Plantenga et al., 2006).

Studies have shown that the 'pungent' aftertaste sensation of piperine is thought to occur via TRPV1, a thermosensor. Piperine is considered to be sharing a common binding site on the vanilloid receptors with other natural compounds like capsaicin and resiniferatoxin.

It has been found that involvement of TRPV1 in broad range of pharmacological/physiological functions is because of its sensitivity to mechanical and thermal stimuli. Hence, effect of piperine on the human vanilloid receptor TRPV1 expressed in HEK293 cells was evaluated by McNamara *et al*. Agonist activity of piperine at TRPV1 was confirmed when it produced a rapidly activating whole-cell currents compared to capsaicin, which were antagonized by capsazepine, a competitive TRPV1 antagonist, and ruthenium red, a non-competitive TRPV1 blocker.

Additionally, a greater degree of efficacy (2-fold larger) than capsaicin in activating TRPV1 was observed. Piperine was also found to induce profound microscopic desensitization of TRPV1 receptor and tachyphylaxis than capsaicin. Overall, it was suggested that piperine exhibits similar effects at human TRPV1 as that of capsaicin, except for a propensity to induce greater receptor desensitization as well as 2-fold higher efficacy than capsaicin itself. Thus, TRPV1-mediated effects of piperine could be of importance in understanding its influence on gastrointestinal function (McNamara et al., 2005).

Effect of vanilloid drugs like anandamide, capsaicin and piperine, which activate vanilloid receptors on gastrointestinal motility was studied *in vivo*. A dose-dependent reduction of upper gastrointestinal transit by piperine was seen. This inhibitory effect of piperine

(10 mg/kg) was significantly attenuated in mice treated with capsaicin (75 mg/kg in total) (Srinivasan, 2009).

In addition, the thermogenic effect of piperine appears to be the result of influence on mitochondrial functions, including the inhibition of oxidative phosphorylation, accumulation and retention of calcium ions and the stimulation of ATPase activity (Westerterp-Plantenga et al., 2006).

Given that thermogenesis is linked to body metabolism and the metabolic rate, there is a high likelihood that piperine-mediated thermoregulation denotes regulation of metabolization of nutrients and drugs. Thus, in view of piperine's influence on multi-mechanism-based nutrient absorption, especially when ingested orally, that too at a dose as little as 5 mg, it is worthy of being termed as a 'supernutrient'. Owing to its potential thermogenic effect on the body, it can also be designated as a 'thermonutrient' (Majeed et al., 1999).

However, it should be noted that thermonutrient does not necessarily corresponds to thermogenic compound. The term *'thermonutirent'* corresponds to a property of a compound to enhance the process of nutrition absorption by enhancing the metabolic process by generating thermal energy (i.e. thermogenesis), whereas the latter term is used to describe a product that is used to increase the heat in the body and in turn, affect the body's metabolism and ability to burn fat (Majeed et al., 1999).

Quantum Chemical and Molecular Docking Techniques:
New Insights into Bioenhancement Property of Piperine

By now, it is understood that piperine enhances bioavailability of several bioactives by inhibiting enzymes, such as UDP-GDH, UGT and cytochrome P450 3A4 (CYP3A4), thereby improving their absorption in the intestine. However, until recently, exact mechanism responsible for this characteristic nature of piperine was not known.

Recent high-level quantum chemical studies coupled with molecular docking techniques have been able to provide new insight into enhanced bioavailability of various agents by piperine, including curcumin.

In the current study, quantum chemical computational analysis followed by set of molecular docking studies between piperine and curcumin, CYP3A4, P-gp and UDP-GDH, and UGT were carried out to understand the mechanisms involved in piperine's role in enhancing bioavailability of curcumin.

Following observations were made from the outcome data:

- Proposed bioenhancement of curcumin (as high as 20-fold; Shoba *et al.*, 1998) by piperine could be due to dual mechanism (Patil *et al.*, 2016):

    - **First Mechanism:** Intercalating propensity of piperine to bind with adjacent layers of curcumin, thus acting as a carrier of curcumin in transporting it through metabolic pathways—thereby increasing curcumin's bioavailability

    - **Second Mechanism:** Piperine inhibits the enzymes responsible for glucuronidation (i.e. CYP3A4, UDP-GDH and UGT) by binding to multiple sites, thereby allowing greater time for the intestine to absorb curcumin

- These observations were further corroborated by molecular docking study, wherein piperine was found to inhibit P-gp, and CYP3A4 and UGT by binding at the nucleotide binding domain and at the transmembrane domain, respectively

Collectively, all of these observations establish that piperine enhances bioavailability of various agents by possessing dual mechanism, i.e. through formation of an intercalation complex as well as by inhibiting enzymes responsible for glucuronidation (e.g. curcumin) (Patil *et al.*, 2016).

Another recently published study by Zeng *et al.* also supports the fact that a time-dependent, selective and reversible inhibition of hepatic and intestinal enzymes involved in curcumin metabolism, such as UGT1A1, 1A6, 1A8, sulfotransferase (SULT) 1A1 and 1A3 may be the novel and alternative mechanism of the bioavailability-enhancing potential of piperine.

In vivo results suggested improved bioavailability of curcumin upon piperine pretreatment was due to rapid inhibition of curcumin metabolism in the absorption phase and not in the elimination phase, which was evident from unaltered T_{max}, $t_{1/2}$ and increased C_{max} of curcumin. Similar results were seen *in vitro*, wherein piperine inhibited most of the UGTs and SULTs in a time-dependent manner in Caco-2 and HepG2 cells. It was concluded that piperine pretreatment exhibits bioenhancing effect on curcumin in a time-dependent, reversible and selective manner (Zeng *et al.*, 2017).

Overall, in the current medical practice, role of bioavailability enhancers has been of clinical significance with profound influence in terms of pharmacokinetic and pharmacodynamic alterations of both prescribed and alternative medicines. Thus, compounds like piperine are considered as one of the most promising bioavailability enhancers to date, which have a great impact on the bioavailability of a broad range of nutritional ingredients.

Chapter 3
Bioavailability Enhancer

Optimum nutrition is key to healthy being, as unhealthy changes in lifestyle and dietary habits have been recognized as primary reasons for several chronic diseases. Effectiveness of nutrients depends on how well they are absorbed, transported, assimilated and reach target organs with minimal biotransformation. In other words, bioavailability of a nutrient is one of the major factors that determine its effectiveness in the human body.

As mentioned earlier (p. 16), *bioenhancer* is an agent capable of enhancing the bioavailability and efficacy of a nutrient with which it is co-administered (Atal and Bedi, 2010).

In Ayurveda, the concept of bioenhancer is mentioned as "*Yogvahi*" (synergism), i.e. increased bioavailability, tissue distribution and efficacy of nutrients/drugs, even when this idea is new to the modern science (Randhawa et al., 2011).

The theory of bioenhancement can vastly be found in the literature of Ayurveda, for example, a large number of prescriptions have been evaluated for the scientific basis of the use of 'trikatu' (three acrids) from the period between 7th century BCE and 6th century CE. It has been reported that these acrids or any one of these three ingredients have the capacity to enhance the bioavailability of certain bioactives (Dudhatra et al., 2012).

However, in the modern era, it was Bose who first reported in 1929 that long pepper enhanced anti-asthmatic effect of an Ayurvedic formula containing *Adhatoda vasica* (Vasaka) leaves (Randhawa *et al.*, 2011). In a later study, long pepper was found to increase the blood levels of test drug, vasicine, by nearly 233%, while the active ingredient piperine could increase the blood levels of sparteine by more than 100% (Atal *et al.*, 1981). Based on these results the authors, for the first time, proposed that piperine increases bioavailability either by promoting rapid absorption from the gastrointestinal tract or by protecting the drug from being metabolized. Thus, piperine or mixtures containing piperine have shown to increase the bioavailability, blood levels and efficacy of many nutraceuticals and drugs.

Sabinsa's BioPerine®, a standardized extract obtained from the fruits of *Piper nigrum*, contains a minimum 95% piperine. It has been shown to significantly enhance the bioavailability of several supplemented nutrients, such as β-carotene, L-(+)-selenomethionine, Se-methyl-L-selenocysteine, vitamin B6, vitamin C, coenzyme Q10 (CoQ10), curcumin, resveratrol, ginseng and elemental iron through their increased absorption.

Following are the nutritional compounds which may be co-administered with piperine to enhance their bioavailability (Dudhatra *et al.*, 2012) (Table 1):

Class	Examples
Herbal Extracts	*Curcuma longa, Boswellia serrata, Withania somnifera, Gingko biloba, Capsicum annuum*, Bioflavonoids, Resveratrol and others
Water-soluble Vitamins	Vitamin B1, Vitamin B2, Niacinamide, Vitamin B6, Vitamin B12, Folic acid and Vitamin C
Fat-soluble Vitamins	Vitamin A, Vitamin D, Vitamin E, Vitamin K and CoQ10
Amino Acids	Lysine, Isoleucine, Leucine, Threonine, Valine, Tryptophan, Phenylalanine, Methionine, L-(+)-Selenomethionine (LSM) and Se-Methyl-L-Selenocysteine (MSC)
Minerals	Iron, Zinc, Copper, Selenium (LSM and MSC), Magnesium, Potassium, Manganese, Vanadium, Iodine, Calcium and Chromium
Antioxidants	Vitamin A, Vitamin C, Vitamin E, α-carotene, β-carotene, β-Cryptoxanthin, Lycopene, Lutein, Zeaxanthin, Pine bark bioflavonoids complex, Selenium and Zinc

Table 1: Nutritional compounds bioenhanced by piperine.

BioPerine® as a Nutrient Bioavailability Enhancer

I. Preclinical Studies

Several studies have confirmed that BioPerine® significantly improves the bioavailability when co-administered with various compounds, such as curcumin, epigallocatechin gallate, resveratrol, *Panax ginseng*, MSC, emodin, elemental iron, linarin, minerals and branched chain amino acids (BCAAs) in animal models.

BioPerine® and Curcumin
BioPerine® and Resveratrol
BioPerine® and BioIron™ (Organic Elemental Iron)
Piperine and (-)-Epigallocatechin-3-Gallate
Piperine and Minerals
BioPerine® and Se-Methyl-L-Selenocysteine
BioPerine® and Panax ginseng
Piperine and Branched Chain Amino Acids
Piperine and Emodin
Piperine and Linarin

Chapter 3
BIOAVAILABILITY ENHANCER

BioPerine® and Curcumin

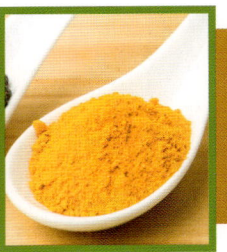

Curcumin derived from the rhizomes of *Curcuma longa* is being used as a dietary supplement and possesses a spectrum of biological and pharmacological activities. It has been a traditional medicine for treating various health conditions. Despite its favorable efficacy and safety profile, low bioavailability and rapid biotransformation have hampered its application as a therapeutic agent. Piperine could improve the uptake of curcumin with clinically validated efficacy in various conditions, including inflammation, cancer, diabetes, metabolic syndrome, arthritis and several other diseases.

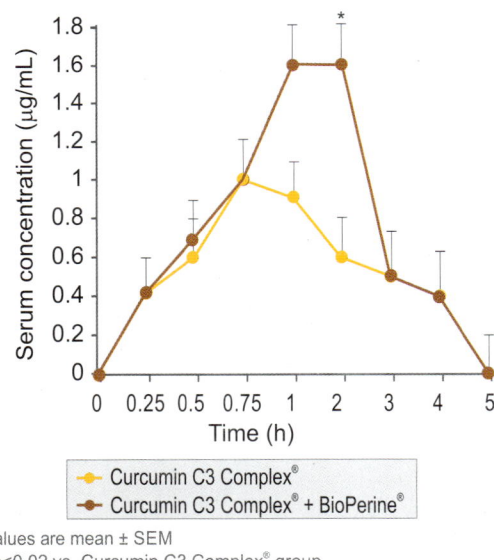

Values are mean ± SEM
*$p<0.02$ vs. Curcumin C3 Complex® group

Fig. 5: Effect of BioPerine® on serum concentrations of Curcumin C3 Complex® in rats.

A rodent study was carried out at St. John's Medical College, Bangalore, India to assess the potential of BioPerine® in increasing the bioavailability of Curcumin C3 Complex®, a versatile phytonutrient obtained from turmeric. Results from the study clearly mentioned that Curcumin C3 Complex® at a dose of 2 g/kg showed moderate serum concentrations over a period of 4 h. However, upon administration of BioPerine® (20 mg/kg), the serum concentration of Curcumin C3 Complex® was increased significantly (Fig. 5) within a short period of time (i.e. 1–2 h) (Shoba *et al.*, 1998).

In another study by Ryu *et al.*, initial brain uptake of fluoropropyl-substituted curcumin (0.77% ID/g at 2 min.) was increased by 48% after co-injecting with piperine when compared to the group without piperine. The fluoropropyl-substituted curcumin group was metabolically stable in the brain and could strongly bind to β-amyloid (Aβ) plaques (Table 2).

(A)

Organ	2 min.	30 min.	60 min.
Brain	0.52 ± 0.08	0.11 ± 0.03	0.11 ± 0.02

(B)

Organ	2 min.	30 min.	60 min.	120 min.
Brain	0.77 ± 0.10	0.14 ± 0.02	0.09 ± 0.02	0.07 ± 0.02

Table 2: Biodistribution of (A) Fluoropropyl-substituted curcumin and (B) Fluoropropyl-substituted curcumin with piperine.

Thus, curcumin derivatives showed higher binding affinities for Aβ aggregates, with fluoropropyl-substituted curcumin being the most potent ligand in normal mice (Ryu et al., 2006).

In another animal model of chronic unpredictable stress (CUS) induced depression, combination of curcumin (20 and 40 mg/kg; i.p., 21 days) with piperine (2.5 mg/kg; i.p., 21 days), showed a significant antidepressant activity in terms of behavioral, biochemical and neurochemical changes when compared to curcumin alone (Bhutani et al., 2009). Piperine co-administration was found to potentiate the neuroprotective activity of curcumin in lipopolysaccharide (LPS) induced depression- and anxiety-like symptoms in mice (Jangra et al., 2016). Better neuroprotective effects were seen against symptoms of Huntington's disease in rats injected with toxins like 3-nitropropionic acid (3-NP) and quinolinic acid (QA) when curcumin was combined with piperine (Singh et al., 2015; Singh and Kumar, 2016).

Kundu et al. also reported that curcumin and piperine-loaded nanoparticles led to improved bioavailability and penetration of curcumin in the brain tissue by crossing the blood brain barrier and thus enhanced neuroprotection in rotenone-induced model of Parkinson's disease (Kundu et al., 2016).

According to Banji et al., combination of piperine and curcumin, the two powerful antioxidants, could reduce the risk of developing neurodegenerative disorders by inhibiting the damage caused by chronic exposure to D-galactose. Additionally, synergistic attenuation of D-galactose-induced senescence in animal model was observed in terms of improved spatial memory, reduced oxidative burden, and improvement in signaling, increase in hippocampal volume and protection of hippocampal neurons (Banji *et al.*, 2013a; 2013b).

The effect of curcumin and piperine in preventing cholesterol gallstone formation was studied in susceptible mice by Li *et al*. The combination decreased the serum cholesterol and triglyceride (TG) levels, reduced the incidence of gallstones by 70% (Table 3) and decreased the expression of Niemann-Pick C1-like 1 (NPC1L1) and sterol response element-binding protein 2 (SREBP2) in both mRNA and protein levels (Li *et al.*, 2015a).

	Length (mm)	Width (mm)	Volume (μL)
Control diet	6.35 ± 0.91	2.75 ± 0.32	25.24 ± 5.97
Lithogenic diet (LD)	8.19 ± 1.71	3.87 ± 0.48	65.54 ± 22.69*
LD + Curcumin (500 mg/kg)	7.91 ± 0.87	3.66 ± 0.50	61.41 ± 18.44
LD + Curcumin (500 mg/kg) + Piperine (20 mg/kg)	6.66 ± 1.36	3.09 ± 0.57	35.98 ± 15.27**

Values are mean ± SD; *p<0.001 vs. Control diet group; **p<0.05 vs. Lithogenic diet group

Table 3: Effect of piperine administration on gallbladder.

In an *in vitro* model, combination of piperine and curcumin completely suppressed the osteoclastogenesis by decreasing the tartrate-resistant acid phosphatase (TRAP) activity (Fig. 6). Combination also inhibited the expression of specific osteoclast markers like TRAP, cathepsin K and calcitonin receptor (Fig. 7) without causing cytotoxic effects in periodontal ligament cells. Thus, combination might act as a bioagent for the prevention and treatment of replacement resorption in replanted teeth (Martins *et al.*, 2015).

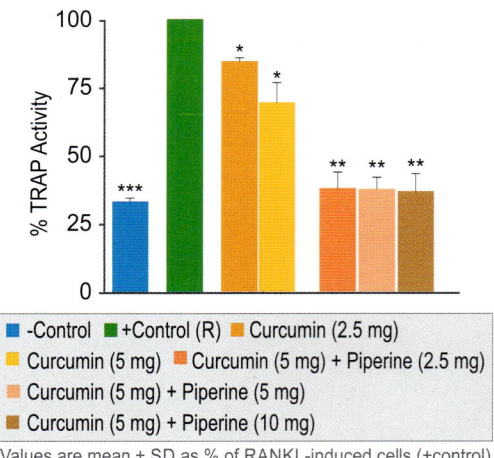

Values are mean ± SD as % of RANKL-induced cells (+control)
*p<0.05, **p<0.001, ***p<0.0001 vs. +Control group

Fig. 6: Influence of piperine and curcumin on TRAP activity.

Chapter 3
BIOAVAILABILITY ENHANCER

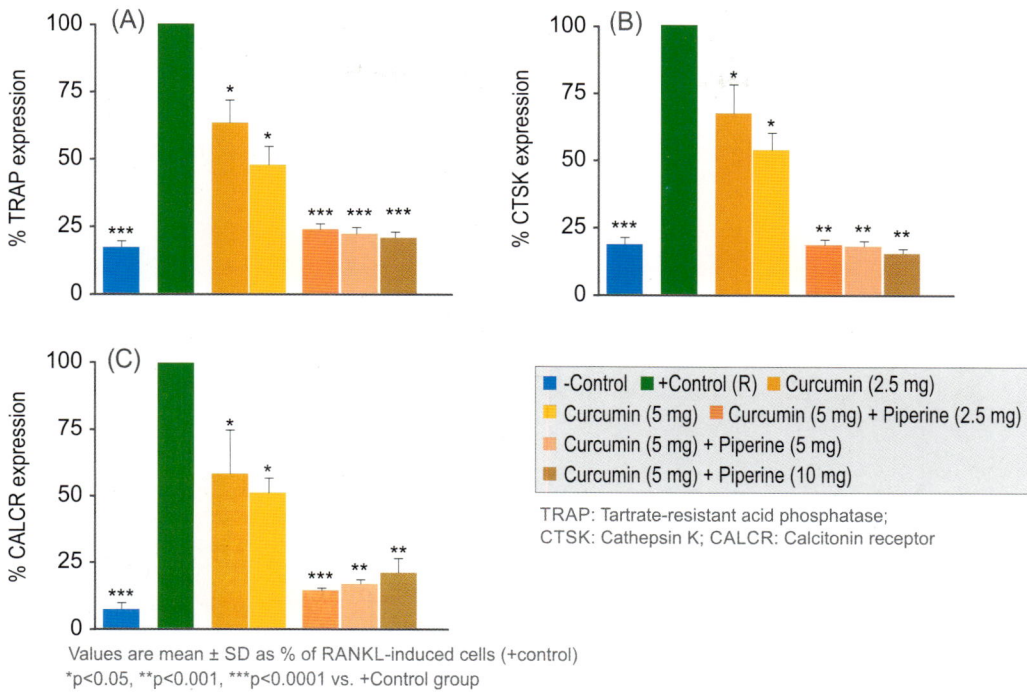

Fig. 7: Effect of curcumin and piperine on the expression of osteoclast gene markers.

In another animal study, treatment with combination of curcumin (100 mg/kg) and piperine (20 mg/kg) for 4 weeks significantly attenuated the morphological, histopathological, biochemical, apoptotic and proliferative changes in the serum and liver of animals with diethylnitrosamine (DENA) induced hepatocellular carcinoma when compared to curcumin alone (Patial et al., 2015).

Suresh and Srinivasan reported that enhanced bioavailability of curcumin (500 mg/kg) was observed in different tissues when co-administered with piperine (20 mg/kg) (Suresh and Srinivasan, 2010).

In an *in vitro* permeability model having Caco-2 cells, increased permeability of curcumin (1.85 ± 0.13) was witnessed when combined with resveratrol and quercetin. However, upon addition of piperine, the permeability further increased to 2.26 ± 0.21. Also curcumin and piperine combination resulted in a permeability increase of 2.33 ± 0.12 when compared to

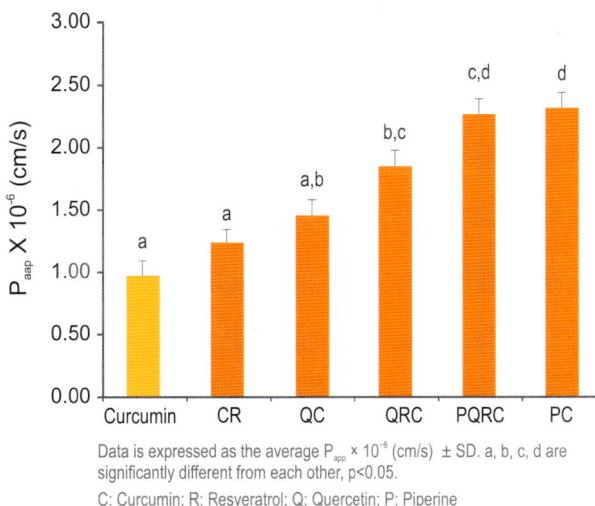

Fig. 8: Influence of piperine and curcumin on apical-to-basal permeability.

Data is expressed as the average $P_{app} \times 10^{-6}$ (cm/s) ± SD. a, b, c, d are significantly different from each other, p<0.05.
C: Curcumin; R: Resveratrol; Q: Quercetin; P: Piperine

curcumin alone (Fig. 8). Thus, piperine appears to have a positive effect on apical-to-basal permeability of curcumin (Lund and Pantuso, 2014).

Significant improvement in glucose tolerance was observed when piperine and quercetin were used to increase the bioavailability of curcumin (Kaur et al., 2016).

In a recent study, Patil et al. using quantum chemical and docking techniques showed that piperine enhances bioavailability of curcumin. The enhanced bioavailability was found to be due to inhibition of enzymes by piperine that cause glucuronidation of curcumin and also through intercalation into curcumin layers through intermolecular hydrogen bonding (Patil et al., 2016).

In another recently published study, bioenhancing activity of piperine as well as the underlying mechanism was evaluated both *in vitro* and *in vivo*. For *in vivo* pharmacokinetic studies, male SD rats were pretreated with piperine (20 mg/kg) at different time points (0.5–8 h) prior to curcumin (200 mg/kg) administration.

Results suggested a significant increase in curcumin exposure in all the piperine pretreated groups, particularly at 6 h, which was evident from significantly higher (p<0.001) C_{max} and AUC_{0-t} (6.09-fold and 5.97-fold increase, respectively), while no change in $t_{1/2}$ and T_{max} was witnessed (Table 4). Piperine was able to inhibit curcumin metabolism in the absorption phase but did not affect in the elimination phase. Thus, it was concluded that increased C_{max} and enhanced bioavailability of curcumin was primarily due to reduced metabolism and not because of altered intestinal absorption rate or prolonged absorption.

Parameter	Curcumin alone (200 mg/kg)	Curcumin (200 mg/kg) + Piperine (20 mg/kg) Co-administration	Curcumin (200 mg/kg) + Piperine (10 mg/kg)				
			Piperine Pretreatment				
			0.5 h	2 h	4 h	6 h	8 h
AUC_{0-t} (µg/l·h)	41.66 ± 12.51	88.95 ± 32.55	167.81 ± 36.37**	114.72 ± 48.84*	132.74 ± 44.57*	228.67 ± 60.87**	126.46 ± 28.04*
$t_{1/2}$ (h)	2.53 ± 1.61	1.98 ± 1.68	2.02 ± 1.22	1.85 ± 0.67	2.99 ± 2.09	1.68 ± 0.83	1.93 ± 1.54
T_{max} (h)	0.12 ± 0.08	0.28 ± 0.21	0.38 ± 0.29	0.12 ± 0.08	0.22 ± 0.08	0.12 ± 0.08	0.22 ± 0.08
C_{max} (µg/l)	59.90 ± 11.37	74.86 ± 21.45	82.59 ± 19.41	76.11 ± 38.36	99.26 ± 26.42	342.93 ± 31.89**	97.12 ± 18.64

Values are mean ± SD; *p<0.05, **p<0.01 vs. Curcumin alone group.
AUC: Area under the curve; $t_{1/2}$: Elimination half-time; T_{max}: Time to reach the maximum plasma concentration; C_{max}: Concentration maximum

Table 4: Influence of piperine pretreatment on pharmacokinetic parameters of curcumin.

Additionally, inhibition of hepatic and intestinal enzymes, such as UGT1A1, 1A6, 1A8, sulfotransferase (SULT) 1A1 and 1A3, which was seen within 6 h of piperine pretreatment was found to be reversed at 8 h. Similar results were obtained when Caco-2 and HepG2 cells were pretreated with piperine *in vitro*. Overall, it was suggested that pretreatment with piperine improves bioavailability of curcumin via reversible and selective inhibition of UGTs and SULTs—a novel and alternative mechanism of the bioavailability-enhancing potential of piperine (Zeng *et al.*, 2017). Based on these observations, it can be said that regulatory effect of piperine is reversible in the short-term with no potent effects.

Chapter 3
BIOAVAILABILITY ENHANCER

BioPerine® and Resveratrol

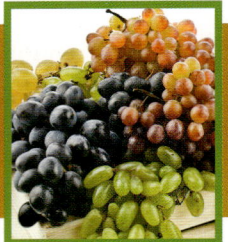

Resveratrol, a naturally occurring phytoalexin found in grapes, berries and many other plants has been shown to possess a large number of health-promoting properties in preclinical studies.

Although laboratory studies have offered a great promise in potential therapeutic and preventative applications, poor bioavailability of resveratrol in formulations has precluded its applicability in controlled clinical settings.

Pharmacokinetic studies in animals and humans have identified that major metabolites of *trans*-resveratrol are derived by glucuronidation or sulfation, and the metabolism of resveratrol has been shown to be very rapid with the majority of biotransformation occurring within the first hour following oral administration. Furthermore, resveratrol metabolites have very short $t_{1/2}$ and are subjected to rapid urinary elimination (Johnson et al., 2011).

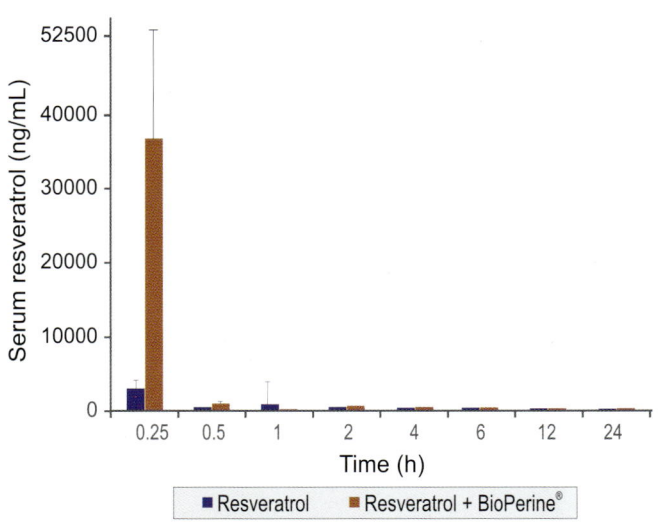

Fig. 9: Effect of BioPerine® on serum concentrations of resveratrol.

The effect of BioPerine® on the absorption and bioavailability of resveratrol was recently studied at University of Wisconsin, USA, using an animal model. Co-administration of BioPerine® (10 mg/kg) significantly improved the bioavailability of resveratrol (100 mg/kg) by 229% and the serum concentration (C_{max}) was increased by 1544% between 0.25 h and 0.5 h. Thus, BioPerine® significantly improved the *in vivo* bioavailability of resveratrol (Fig. 9). The current study signifies that inhibition of glucuronidation of resveratrol by BioPerine® resulted in its improved bioavailability (Johnson et al., 2011).

In another study, combination of *trans*-resveratrol with piperine reduced the immobility time of rats when compared to *trans*-resveratrol alone and thus, could act as an alternative therapy by providing protection against chronic stress (Xu et al., 2016).

Chapter 3
BIOAVAILABILITY ENHANCER

BioPerine® and BioIron™ (Organic Elemental Iron)

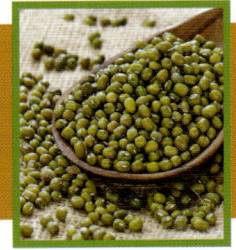

Iron, an essential trace mineral, plays a vital role in oxygen transport, oxidative metabolism, cellular proliferation and many other physiological processes. One of the foremost health concerns worldwide is the deficiency of iron, primarily being poor bioavailability or poor dietary intake.

BioIron™, a naturally enriched source of elemental iron, is obtained from mung beans (green gram) by a soil-less process through the technology of hydroponics.

An *in vivo* study was performed to evaluate the bioavailability of organic elemental iron (BioIron™) in combination with or without BioPerine®. A single oral dose of BioIron™ with or without BioPerine® was supplemented to rabbits. Results showed that at 8 h time point serum concentration of iron was significantly higher in group treated with BioIron™ containing BioPerine® (36.55 ± 9.97 µg/ml) when compared to the group without BioPerine® (Fig. 10) (Majeed *et al.*, 2016a).

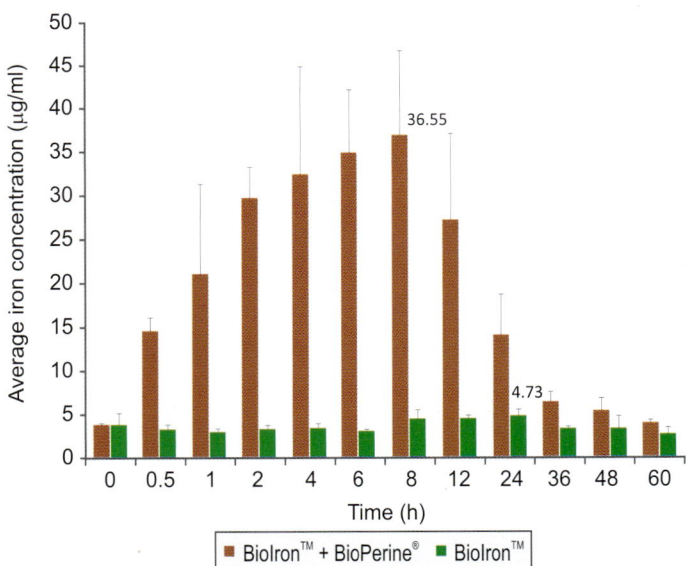

Fig. 10: Effect of BioPerine® on serum concentration of BioIron™.

Chapter 3
BIOAVAILABILITY ENHANCER

Piperine and (-)-Epigallocatechin-3-Gallate

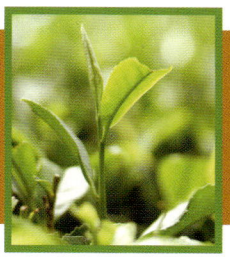

Piperine has been reported to enhance the bioavailability of tea polyphenol (-)-epigallocatechin-3-gallate (EGCG) in an animal model. When piperine (70.2 µmol/kg) was co-administered with EGCG (163.8 µmol/kg; i.g.) to male CF-1 mice, plasma levels of total and unconjugated EGCG increased by 1.1- and 1.4-fold, respectively, while area under curve (AUC) increased by 1.2- and 1.3-fold, respectively compared to EGCG group.

	C_{max}		AUC_{60-300}	
	EGCG	EGCG + Piperine	EGCG	EGCG + Piperine
Plasma	µmol/L		µmol/L•min.	
i. Unconjugated	0.05 ± 0.01	0.12 ± 0.04*	9.95 ± 1.09	22.67 ± 4.18*
ii. Total	0.32 ± 0.05	0.66 ± 0.16*	53.82 ± 7.95	118.71 ± 24.99*
	nmol/g		nmol/g•min.	
Small intestine, total[#]	37.50 ± 22.50	31.60 ± 15.68	1686.50 ± 757.07	4621.80 ± 1958.72*
Colon, total[#]	3.76 ± 1.93	0.47 ± 0.14*	325.10 ± 109.58	85.20 ± 25.44*

Values are mean ± SEM; *$p<0.01$ vs. EGCG group. [#]All unconjugated | C_{max}: Maximum plasma concentration; AUC: Area under the curve

Table 5: Effect of piperine on AUC and C_{max} of EGCG in the plasma and tissues of mice.

The levels of EGCG in the small intestine remained higher for a longer period of time following piperine treatment (C_{max} = 31.60 ± 15.08 nmol/g at 90 min. and levels were maintained above 20 nmol/g until 180 min.) compared to the group treated with EGCG alone (Table 5). The appearance of EGCG level in the colon and feces were lower than that in mice treated with EGCG alone (Fig. 11). Piperine (100 µM) was found to inhibit EGCG glucuronidation in the small intestine of mice by 40%. Piperine was also found to inhibit the production of EGCG-3''-glucuronide in human HT-29 colon carcinoma cells.

Chapter 3
BIOAVAILABILITY ENHANCER

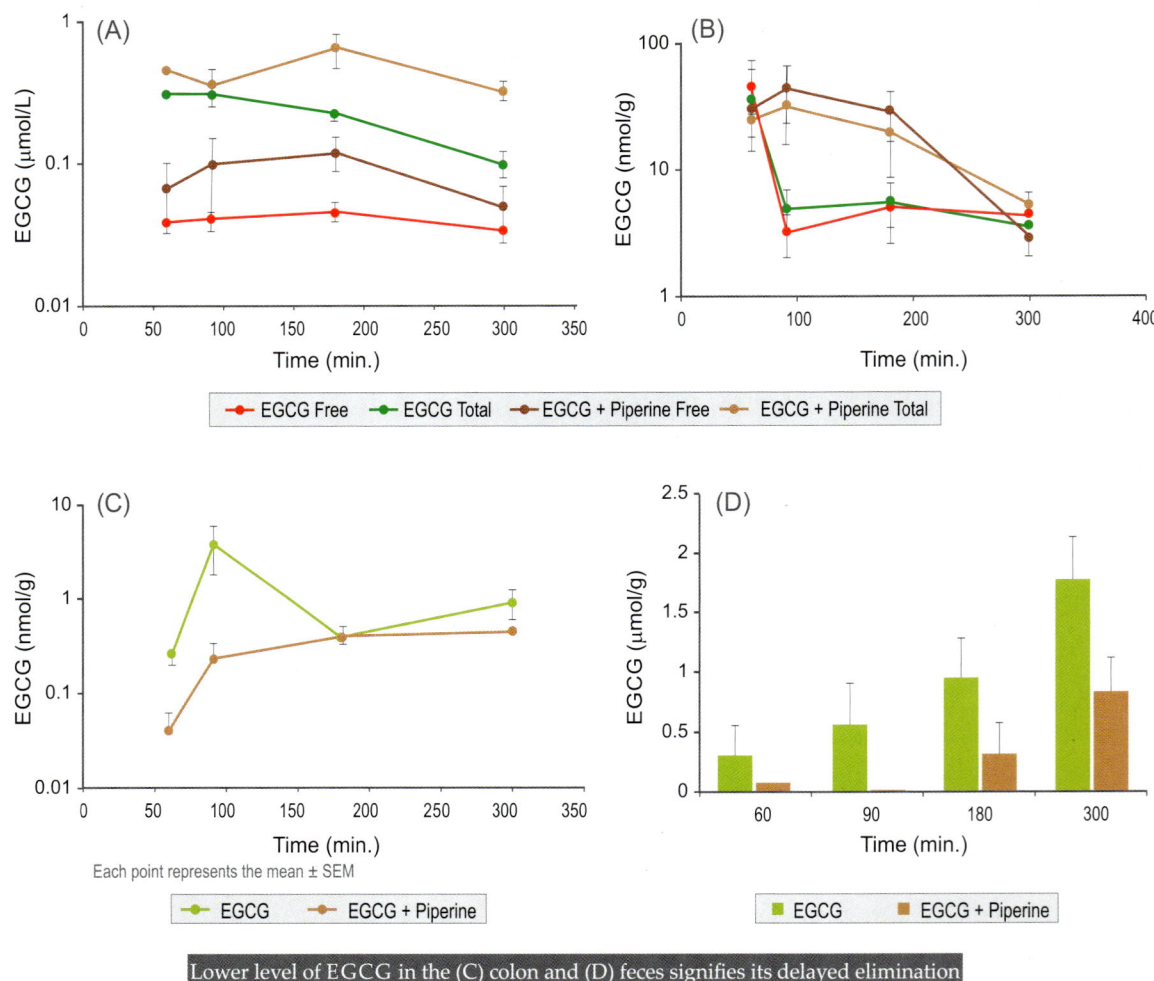

Fig. 11: Influence of piperine on EGCG levels of (A) Plasma (B) Small intestine (C) Colon (D) Feces.

In conclusion, piperine increased EGCG bioavailability by inhibiting glucuronidation and slowing the gastrointestinal transit, thus increasing the residence time in the intestine—resulting in greater absorption (Lambert *et al.*, 2004).

Chapter 3
BIOAVAILABILITY ENHANCER

Piperine and Minerals

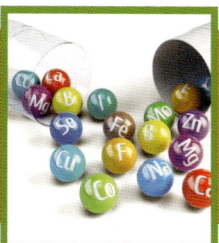

Piperine and other spices (capsaicin, ginger) were studied in an animal model for their influence on absorption of minerals, such as calcium, iron and zinc.

Everted segments of small intestines (i.e. duodenum, jejunum and ileum portions) isolated from rats fed with piperine and other spices were examined for the uptake of iron, zinc and calcium *ex vivo* present in the incubation medium containing digesta of finger millet flour or fortified finger millet flour.

The study found that piperine's bioenhancing effect was the highest for calcium when compared to those of iron and zinc (Table 6A and 6B). Based on the results, authors suggested that piperine enhances bioavailability either by promoting rapid absorption from the gut or by retarding metabolism by the liver or a combination of these two mechanisms (Prakash and Srinivasan, 2013).

Diet Group	(A) Digesta of finger millet flour			
	Intestinal uptake of calcium (µg/g tissue/30 min.)		Percent of calcium uptake from the incubation medium	
	Jejunum	Ileum	Jejunum	Ileum
Control	22.1 ± 0.36	22.5 ± 0.29	8.07 ± 0.17	8.36 ± 0.34
Capsaicin	31.6 ± 1.22*	30.6 ± 0.53*	9.72 ± 0.23*	10.2 ± 0.80*
Piperine	46.4 ± 2.35*	42.6 ± 1.43*	16.1 ± 1.15*	14.2 ± 0.73*
Ginger	43.9 ± 1.80*	40.1 ± 6.33*	14.3 ± 1.47*	13.3 ± 1.03*

Values are mean ± SEM; *$p<0.05$ vs. Control group

Diet Group	(B) Digesta of fortified finger millet flour					
	Intestinal uptake of calcium (µg/g tissue/30 min.)			Percent of calcium uptake from the incubation medium		
	Duodenum	Jejunum	Ileum	Duodenum	Jejunum	Ileum
Control	13.3 ± 1.65	13.1 ± 0.28	15.6 ± 0.73	5.42 ± 0.79	5.10 ± 0.65	5.69 ± 0.43
Capsaicin	29.7 ± 1.73*	22.5 ± 1.00*	24.7 ± 1.76*	8.59 ± 0.56*	6.93 ± 0.26*	7.34 ± 0.22*
Piperine	31.6 ± 1.57*	30.3 ± 1.99*	27.4 ± 1.63*	10.7 ± 1.21*	9.26 ± 0.88*	14.0 ± 0.73*
Ginger	31.7 ± 2.90*	30.3 ± 0.82*	30.8 ± 1.25*	11.9 ± 1.06*	14.1 ± 1.33*	12.1 ± 0.82*

Values are mean ± SEM; *$p<0.05$ vs. Control group

Table 6: Uptake of calcium from the digesta of (A) Finger millet (B) Fortified finger millet flour.

Chapter 3
BIOAVAILABILITY ENHANCER

BioPerine® and Se-Methyl-L-Selenocysteine

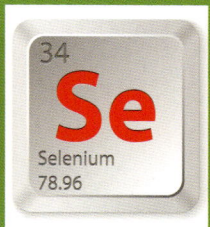

Selenium is an essential trace nutrient with multiple roles in growth and functioning of living cells in higher animals and humans. Se-methyl-L-selenocysteine, this form of selenium has been extensively researched in recent years as a safe and bioavailable form of supplemental dietary selenium.

In an animal study, when Se-methyl-L-selenocysteine was co-administered with BioPerine®, it showed superior efficacy and safety in suppressing macrophage-associated liver injury and endotoxemia when compared to the group without BioPerine®, thus showing enhanced bioavailability (Table 7) (Majeed *et al.*, 2006).

Parameter	Treatment			
	Control (Normal)	Control (*P. acnes* + LPS)	Se-Methyl-L-Selenocysteine Treated	Se-Methyl-L-Selenocysteine + BioPerine® Treated
TNF-α (ng/ml)	40 ± 3	92 ± 4	81 ± 6	55 ± 4**
Serum lipid peroxides (MDA formed/mg protein)	2.35 ± 0.21	3.83 ± 0.33	2.71 ± 0.32	2.59 ± 0.25**
SOD (Units/min./mg protein)	5.62 ± 0.46	3.97 ± 0.41	4.91 ± 0.48	5.57 ± 0.50**
Catalase (μM of H_2O_2 consumed/min./mg protein)	47.12 ± 4.30	22.16 ± 2.07	31.16 ± 3.95	45.07 ± 4.23**
Glutathione peroxidase (μM of GSH oxidized/min./mg protein)	9.23 ± 0.82	5.78 ± 0.53	8.13 ± 0.71	9.08 ± 0.85**
GSH (μg/mg protein)	8.65 ± 0.72	6.16 ± 0.56	7.43 ± 0.69	8.24 ± 0.65**

**$p<0.05$ vs. Control (*P. acnes* + LPS) group

LPS: Lipopolysaccharide; TNF-α: Tumor necrosis factor-alpha; GSH: Glutathione; H_2O_2: Hydrogen peroxide; MDA: Malondialdehyde; SOD: Superoxide dismutase

Table 7: Effect of piperine on the efficacy of Se-methyl-L-selenocysteine.

BioPerine® and Panax ginseng

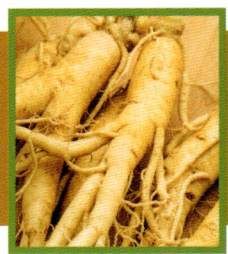

Panax ginseng has been commonly used as an adaptogenic agent and its major bioactive components are ginsenosides, a group of saponins with dammarane triterpenoid structure. Ginsenosides are primarily classified into two major groups, namely protopanaxadiol (PPD) and protopanaxatriol (PPT), based on the type, position and number of sugar moieties attached by the glycosidic bonds. The PPD type includes ginsenosides Rb1, Rb2, Rc, and Rd and rare types Rg3 and Rh2, where as PPT type includes Re, Rf, Rg1, Rg2 and Rh1 (Popovich *et al.*, 2012).

When orally administered, because of hydrophilic nature of ginseng its main constituents (ginseng saponins and polysaccharides) cannot be easily absorbed from the intestine. As a result, these constituents come into contact with intestinal microflora in the alimentary tract and get metabolized by intestinal microflora. Compound K (20S-protopanaxadiol 20-O-beta-D-glucopyranoside) and 20S-protopanaxatriol are the resulting metabolites, which are then easily absorbed from the gastrointestinal tract because they are non-polar and found to be pharmacologically active (Kim, 2012).

Compound K has been reported to be the major ginsenoside metabolite produced, which can be detected in the urine and blood after administration of ginseng (Kim, 2015). It has been shown to have anti-inflammatory, antioxidant and neuroprotective activities and also reported to induce tumor cell apoptosis, inhibit tumor metastasis and restrain tumor invasion (Popovich *et al.*, 2012). Ginsenosides have been reported to have anticancer, antidiabetic, immunomodulatory functions and also help improve central nervous system (CNS) functions.

In an animal model, co-administration of BioPerine® with *Panax ginseng* was found to maximize the antioxidant effect of saponins, thus claiming bioenhancement of ginseng

Chapter 3
BIOAVAILABILITY ENHANCER

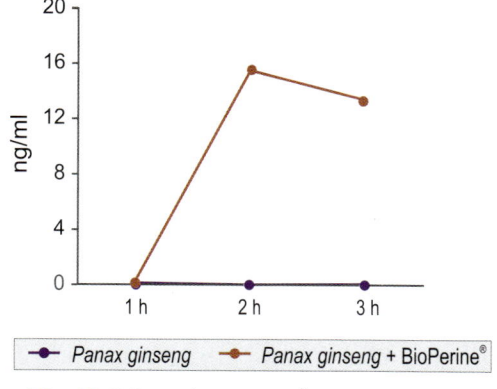

Fig. 12: Effect of BioPerine® on compound K levels with *Panax ginseng*.

saponin. BioPerine® was also found to improve the absorption of compound K compared to ginseng alone group (Fig. 12) (Hee *et al.*, 2013).

In another study, bioavailability of cubic nanoparticles containing PPD along with piperine and PPD nanoparticles alone were compared to free PPD *in vitro* and *in vivo* by Jin *et al.* PPD-cubosome alone and PPD-cubosome loaded with piperine were found to increase the apical-to-basolateral permeability of PPD across the Caco-2 cell monolayer from 53% to 64%, respectively compared to free PPD. The bioavailability of PPD-cubosome and PPD-cubosome loaded with piperine in terms of AUC was increased by 166% and 248%, respectively compared to free PPD (Table 8). Thus, it was thought that piperine possesses inherent anticancer property by improving the oral bioavailability of PPD (Jin *et al.*, 2013).

Parameters	PPD	PPD-cubosome	PPD-cubosome loaded with piperine
AUC_{0-t} (mg/L·min.)	25.76 ± 4.38	43.37 ± 6.39*	64.11 ± 10.28*,#
$AUC_{0-\infty}$ (mg/L·min.)	28.01 ± 4.02	47.44 ± 7.21*	69.53 ± 12.76*,#
MRT_{0-t} (min.)	361.18 ± 51.43	396.18 ± 43.45*	407.12 ± 52.47*
$MRT_{0-\infty}$ (min.)	489.76 ± 63.44	531.79 ± 60.28*	530.17 ± 72.33*
CL (L/min./kg)	0.071 ± 0.028	0.068 ± 0.031	0.029 ± 0.011*,#
$t_{1/2}$ (min.)	324.01 ± 33.49	372.59 ± 49.41	345.93 ± 45.23
T_{max} (min.)	85 ± 20.61	125 ± 29.49*	110 ± 14.14*
C_{max} (ng/mL)	73.45 ± 13.56	100.14 ± 19.40*	142.13 ± 31.11*,#

Data represent the mean ± SD; *p<0.05 vs. PPD; #p<0.05 vs. PPD-cubosome.
AUC: Area under the curve; MRT: Mean residence time; CL: Mean the clearance; $t_{1/2}$: Half life; T_{max}: Time to maximum plasma concentration; C_{max}: Maximum plasma concentration; PPD: 20(S)-Protopanaxadiol

Table 8: Pharmacokinetic parameters of PPD, PPD-cubosome and PPD-cubosome loaded with piperine.

Piperine and Branched Chain Amino Acids

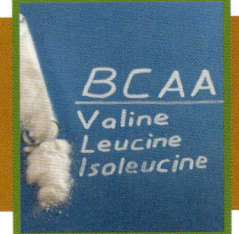

Amino acids are the building blocks of protein and are necessary for nearly every biological process in the body. Among the nine essential amino acids, three are considered to be the branched chain amino acids: leucine, isoleucine and valine, which cannot be synthesized by the body and must be obtained from dietary sources. Branched chain amino acids play an important role in protein synthesis and energy production.

In an *in vitro* study, piperine enhanced the uptake of radiolabelled BCAAs like L-valine, L-leucine and L-isoleucine in epithelial cells when compared to the control (Table 9) (Johri *et al.*, 1992).

[^{14}C] Amino acids	Uptake (pmol/mg protein)			
	Peak		Equilibrium	
	Control	Piperine-treated*	Control†	Piperine-treated†
L- leucine	543 ± 17	680 ± 12	201 ± 11	217 ± 19
L- isoleucine	510 ± 20	695 ± 18	240 ± 17	249 ± 13
L- valine	490 ± 15	610 ± 13	211 ± 13	220 ± 11

Values are mean ± SEM; *p<0.001 vs. Control values at peak time; †p<0.001 vs. Corresponding values at peak time

Table 9: Effect of piperine on the uptake of amino acids in epithelial cells.

Chapter 3
BIOAVAILABILITY ENHANCER

Piperine and Emodin

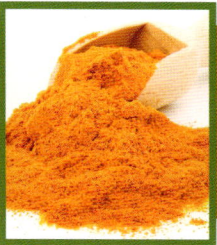

Emodin (1,3,8-trihydroxy-6-methylanthraquinone), an anthraquinone derivative, has been widely used as a traditional medicine and shown to have a large number of health-promoting properties. Due to its low bioavailability piperine was added to enhance the bioavailability of emodin. Results showed that piperine significantly improved the *in vivo* bioavailability by inhibiting its glucuronidation (Fig. 13). Pharmacokinetic parameters (AUC and C_{max}) of emodin were also significantly increased after piperine reatment (Di *et al.*, 2015).

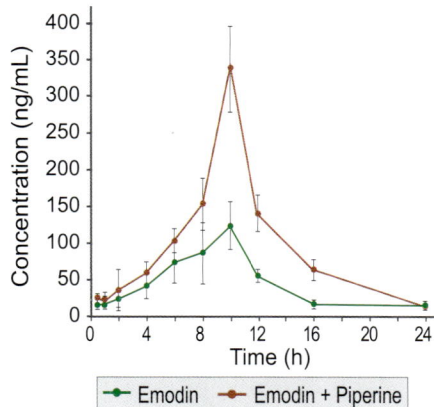

Fig. 13: Mean plasma concentration-time curve of emodin with piperine.

Chapter 3
BIOAVAILABILITY ENHANCER

Piperine and Linarin

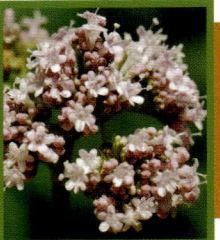

Linarin, a natural flavonoid glycoside, found in *Valeriana officinalis* has been reported to have neuroprotective activities due to its anti-cholinesterase and sleep-enhancing properties (Fernández *et al.*, 2004).

Piperine was found to increase the permeability of linarin significantly as compared to linarin alone (Fig. 14A). Also, co-administration of piperine increased the C_{max} and AUC of linarin by 346% and 381%, respectively (Fig. 14B and Table 10) (Feng *et al.*, 2014).

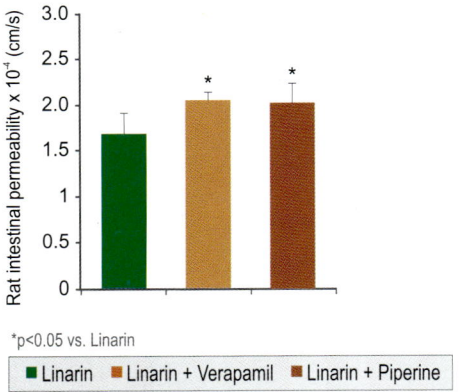

Fig. 14A: Intestinal permeability of piperine with linarin.

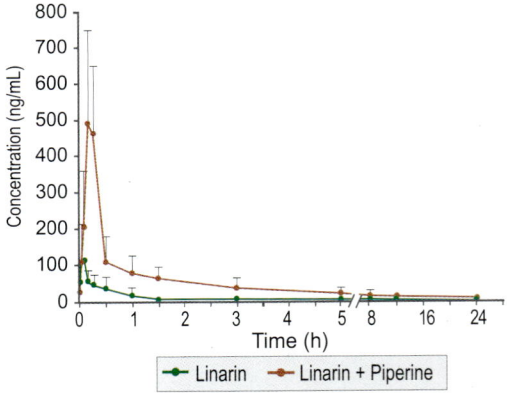

Fig. 14B: Mean plasma concentration-time curve of linarin with piperine.

Parameters	Linarin	Linarin + Piperine
$t_{1/2}$ (h)	4.2 ± 1.3	4.7 ± 2.8
CL_z (L/h/kg)	556 ± 320	118 ± 75
AUC_{0-t} (ng•h/mL)	106 ± 67	554 ± 316
$AUC_{0-\infty}$ (ng•h/mL)	122 ± 76	587 ± 347
T_{max} (h)	0.053 ± 0.027	0.200 ± 0.046
C_{max} (ng/mL)	145 ± 32	647 ± 96

Values are mean ± SD   AUC: Area under the curve; CL_z: Mean the clearance; $t_{1/2}$: Half life; T_{max}: Time to maximum plasma concentration; C_{max}: Maximum plasma concentration

Table 10: Pharmacokinetic parameters of linarin alone and in combination with piperine.

BioPerine® as a Nutrient Bioavailability Enhancer

II. Clinical Studies

Several studies have confirmed that co-administration of BioPerine® has increased the bioavailability of various phytonutrients, minerals and vitamins.

BioPerine® and Curcumin C3 Complex®

BioPerine® and Coenzyme Q10

BioPerine® and β-Carotene

BioPerine® and L-(+)-Selenomethionine

BioPerine® and Se-Methyl-L-Selenocysteine

BioPerine® and Vitamin B6

BioPerine® and Vitamin C with Propranolol Hydrochloride

BioPerine® and Resveratrol

BioPerine® and BioIron™ (Organic Elemental Iron)

Chapter 3
BIOAVAILABILITY ENHANCER

BioPerine® and Curcumin C3 Complex®

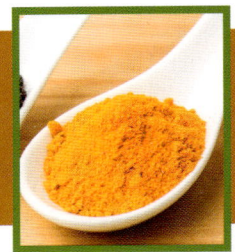

Based on the animal study results (Shoba *et al.*, 1998), a randomized, cross-over, clinical trial was carried out at St. John's Medical College, Bangalore, India to assess the potential of BioPerine® in increasing the bioavailability of Curcumin C3 Complex®.

The subjects were administered 2 g curcumin, followed by two weeks of washout period and crossed over to receive Curcumin C3 Complex® (2 g) and BioPerine® (20 mg) combination. Blood samples were taken at 0.25, 0.5, 0.75, 1, 2, 3, 4, 5 and 6 h post-administration. Both Curcumin C3 Complex® and Curcumin C3 Complex®-BioPerine® combination were well tolerated with no adverse events. Results demonstrated that BioPerine® enhanced the oral bioavailability of Curcumin C3 Complex® with serum concentration of curcumin peaking at 0.75 h and relative bioavailability of curcumin increasing by 2000% or 20 folds (Fig. 15).

This study signifies that BioPerine® is a potent inhibitor of metabolism of certain nutrients/dietary ingredients, which can alter the rate of glucuronidation in the gut and liver, thus slowing down the transformation and increasing the bioavailability in both rats and healthy human volunteers.

This study was a path-breaking and first-of-its-kind to demonstrate bioenhancing potential of BioPerine®, and is one of the most downloaded papers of *Planta Medica* journal* (Shoba *et al.*, 1998).

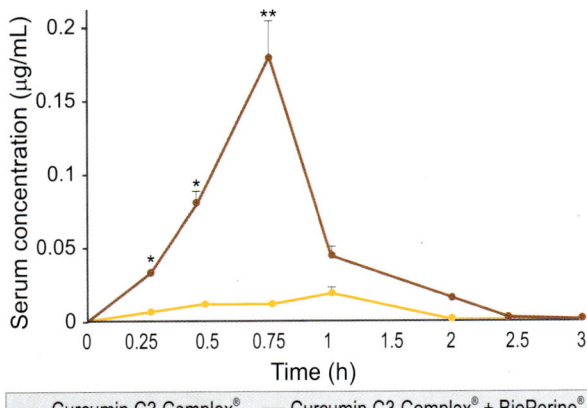

Values are mean ± SEM
*$p<0.01$, **$p<0.001$ vs. Curcumin C3 Complex® group

Fig. 15: Effect of BioPerine® on serum concentrations of Curcumin C3 Complex® in human volunteers.

* https://www.thieme-connect.com/products/ejournals/topten/_plantamedica

Furthermore, researchers have continued to use Curcumin C3 Complex® and BioPerine® combination in a variety of studies and have shown its efficacy in various health conditions, including Alzheimer's disease, cognitive impairment and several types of premalignant and malignant cancers.

In a 30-day, randomized, double-blind, placebo-controlled, cross-over study conducted in Iran, the combination of Curcumin C3 Complex® (1 g) and BioPerine® (10 mg) significantly lowered the TG levels in obese subjects (Mohammadi et al., 2013).

Researchers at Baqiyatallah University of Medical Sciences, Tehran, Iran conducted a clinical trial with Curcumin C3 Complex® and BioPerine® combination for evaluating its role in the management of knee osteoarthritis and showed that BioPerine® can increase the bioavailability without compromising the safety or efficacy of curcuminoids (Panahi et al., 2014). In another study by the same research group, use of Curcumin C3 Complex® and BioPerine® was well tolerated, safe and helped in the managing symptoms of major depressive disorder (Panahi et al., 2015).

Researchers at Mashhad University of Medical Sciences, Mashhad, Iran also conducted a randomized, double-blind, cross-over study to evaluate anxiolytic effects of Curcumin C3 Complex®. Supplementation for 4 weeks in obese subjects was able to show significant anti-anxiety effects. Authors also explained that bioavailability issue of Curcumin C3 Complex® supplementation was overcome by the addition of BioPerine® as a bioavailability enhancer (Esmaily et al., 2015).

In a recent 8-week, randomized, controlled clinical trial, significantly improved antioxidant capacity of Curcumin C3 Complex® (1000 mg/day) in patients with type II diabetes was observed, when co-supplemented with BioPerine® (10 mg/day) (Panahi et al., 2017).

Chapter 3
BIOAVAILABILITY ENHANCER

BioPerine® and Coenzyme Q10

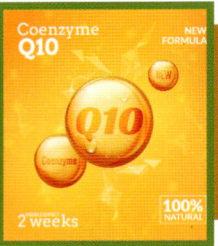

In a double-blind study, relative bioavailability of 90 mg and 120 mg of CoQ10 was evaluated in a single dose experiment or in separate experiments for 14 and 21 days with or without BioPerine® (5 mg) supplementation in 12 healthy adult male volunteers.

Results of single dose and 14-day study showed no significant increase in plasma concentrations of CoQ10 in control compared with group receiving supplement of BioPerine®. However, supplementation of 120 mg of CoQ10 co-administered with BioPerine® for 21 days resulted in absolute increase in blood serum levels of CoQ10 by 1.12 µg/ml vs. 0.85 µg/ml in the control group. Overall, a 30% increase was observed in AUC of CoQ10 when supplemented with BioPerine® compared to control (Fig. 16).

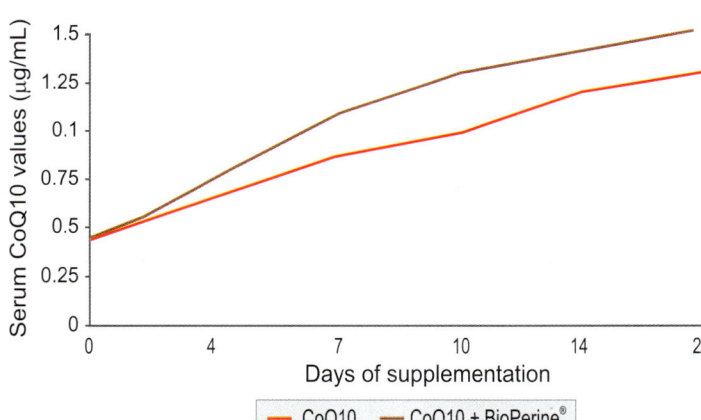

Fig. 16: Effect of BioPerine® on serum CoQ10 levels.

Hence, the present study demonstrated that piperine increases absorption of CoQ10 through its non-specific, thermogenic property. This combined supplementation might be helpful in patients diagnosed with low plasma levels of CoQ10 and in elderly individuals with poor gastrointestinal absorption (Badmaev *et al.*, 2000).

Chapter 3
BIOAVAILABILITY ENHANCER

BioPerine® and β-Carotene

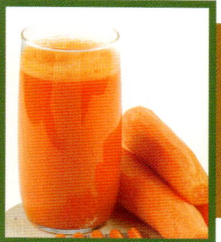

In a double-blind, cross-over study when BioPerine® (5 mg) was combined with β-carotene (15 mg), a fat-soluble vitamin precursor, given as a dietary supplement once a day increased the blood levels of β-carotene in human volunteers almost by 2 folds.

Supplementation with β-carotene plus BioPerine® for 14 days produced a 60% increase in the AUC as compared to β-carotene administered alone (Fig. 17).

It has also been reported that piperine did not alter the levels of retinol—signifying that piperine has no effect on the metabolic pathways of retinol. This study also suggests that bioenhancing mechanism of BioPerine® to increase the oral β-carotene supplementation is through non-specific, thermogenic property (Badmaev et al., 1999).

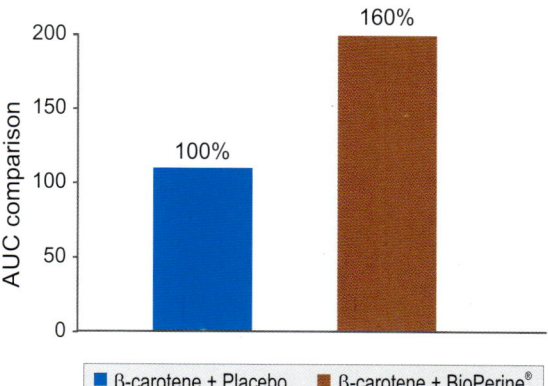

Fig. 17: Effect of BioPerine® on the mean serum β–carotene levels.

Chapter 3
BIOAVAILABILITY ENHANCER

BioPerine® and L-(+)-Selenomethionine

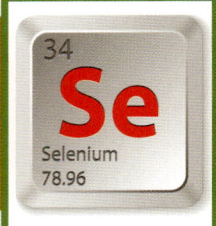

In a double-blind study comprising of 10 subjects, bioavailability of selenium alone [in the form of L-(+)-selenomethionine (50 µg)] and when supplemented with BioPerine® (5 mg) was evaluated over the course of 6 weeks (Fig. 18). The serum selenium levels were approximately 30% higher in the group receiving selenium and BioPerine® after 2 weeks of treatment with a plateau in the subsequent time points tested (Majeed *et al.*, 1999).

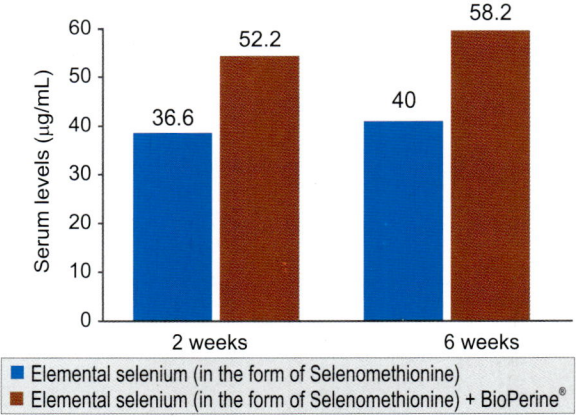

Fig. 18: Effect of BioPerine® on serum selenium levels.

Chapter 3
BIOAVAILABILITY ENHANCER

BioPerine® and Se-Methyl-L-Selenocysteine

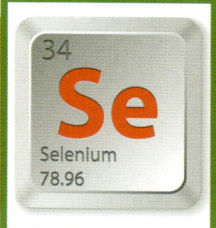

In an open, prospective study, combination of Se-methyl-L-selenocysteine (100 µg of selenium) with BioPerine® (5 mg) showed a reduction in plasma lipid peroxidation level (Fig. 19A), increase in glutathione-S-transferase (GST) (Fig. 19B) and superoxide dismutase (SOD) activities (Fig. 19C), and decrease in the catalase activity (Fig. 19D). Thus, combination of Se-methyl-L-selenocysteine with BioPerine® effectively reduced the oxidative stress levels with statistically significant difference from day 0 (baseline) to day 21 and day 42 (Fig. 19). Hence, this combination was proved to be safe for use as an antioxidant nutritional supplement with enhanced bioavailability (Majeed et al., 2006).

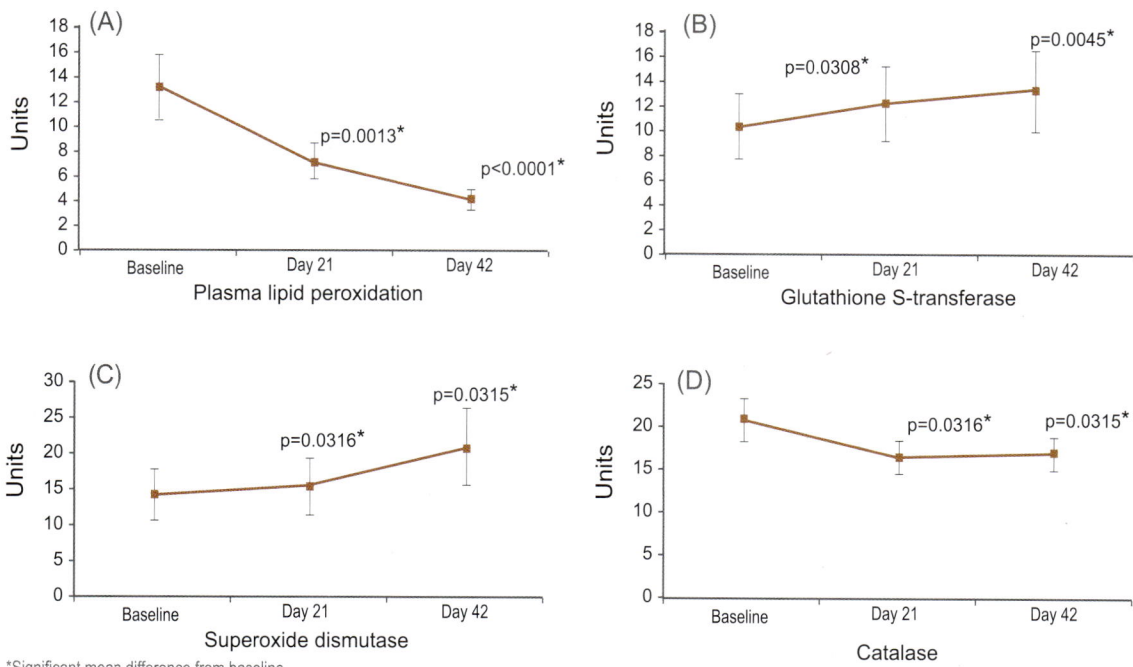

*Significant mean difference from baseline

Fig. 19: Antioxidant activity of Se-methyl-L-selenocysteine with BioPerine®.

BioPerine® and Vitamin B6

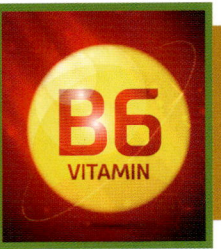

A single dose of 100 mg of vitamin B6 was supplemented to six healthy volunteers and bioavailability was evaluated with and without BioPerine®.

At 2 h, the maximum serum levels of vitamin B6 were 2.5 times higher in the group receiving combination as compared to the control. At 4 h, the concentration of vitamin B6 level in the group receiving vitamin B6 and BioPerine® was 1.4 times higher as compared to the control group (Fig. 20). None of the volunteers complained of any side effects during the study course (Majeed et al., 1999).

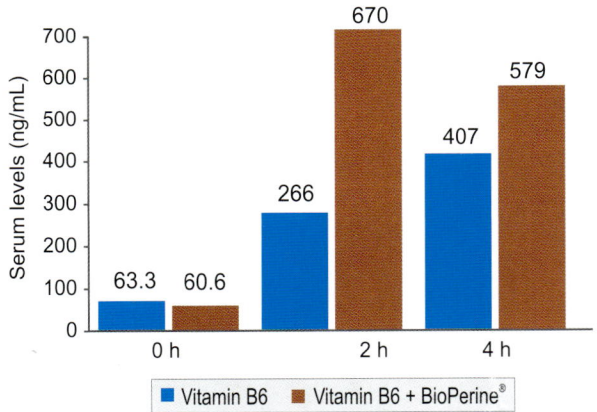

Fig. 20: Effect of BioPerine® on the bioavailability of vitamin B6.

Chapter 3
BIOAVAILABILITY ENHANCER

BioPerine® and Vitamin C with Propranolol Hydrochloride

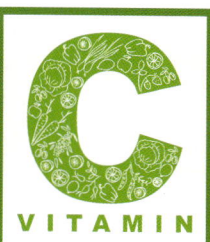

In a double-blind, cross-over study, when BioPerine® (5 mg) was added to a mixture of vitamin C (500 mg) and propranolol hydrochloride (10 mg) bioavailability of the nutrient was enhanced, while that of propranolol's remained unchanged. Thus, presence of BioPerine® resulted in 39.2% increase in vitamin C plasma levels as compared to control levels (Fig. 21). On the other hand, measurement of propanolol hydrochloride plasma levels did not show any significant change (Majeed *et al.*, 1999).

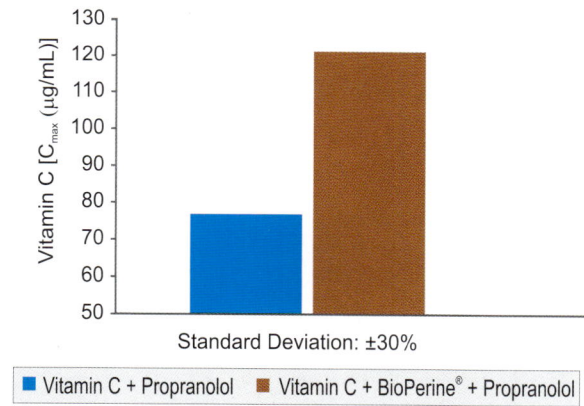

Fig. 21: Effect of BioPerine® on the bioavailability of vitamin C with propranolol.

Chapter 3
BIOAVAILABILITY ENHANCER

BioPerine® and Resveratrol

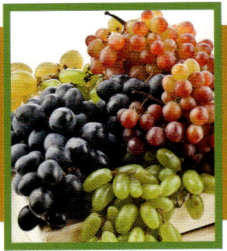

In a double-blind, placebo-controlled, 4-week clinical trial, 16 healthy young adults were recruited, wherein effects of resveratrol (500 mg) and BioPerine® (10 mg) supplementation in combination with exercise training on skeletal muscle mitochondrial performance were evaluated.

All participants performed 3 sessions of sub-maximal endurance training of the wrist flexor muscles of the non-dominant arm every week. The contra-lateral arm served as an untrained control. Study report suggested that combination group showed significant changes in mitochondrial performance from baseline to post-testing (40 % increase) ($\Delta k=0.58$, $p=0.001$) and compared with placebo ($p<0.05$) at week 4 (Fig. 22).

Overall, it was concluded that supplementation with resveratrol and BioPerine® combination might be helpful in enhancing skeletal muscle mitochondrial performance during low-intensity exercise training (Polley *et al.*, 2016).

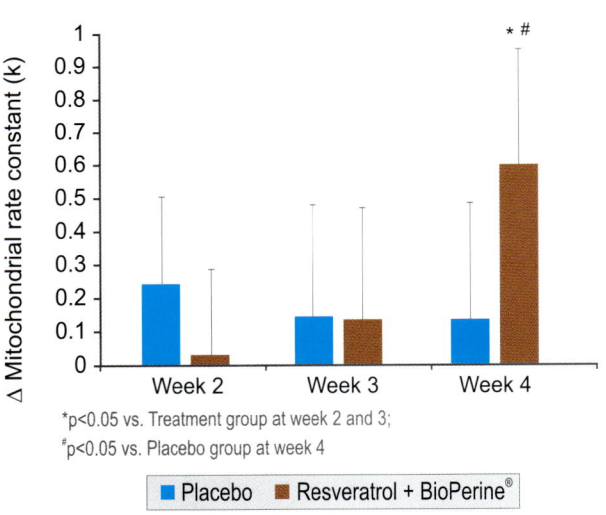

Fig. 22: Effect of resveratrol and BioPerine® combination on change in mitochondrial performance.

Chapter 3
BIOAVAILABILITY ENHANCER

BioPerine® and BioIron™ (Organic Elemental Iron)

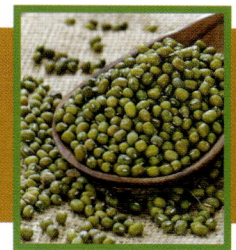

In an open-label, non-randomized study, 30 subjects were provided with BioIron™ tablet (containing 8.5 mg of elemental iron and 2.5 mg of BioPerine®) twice a day as a dietary supplement for a period of 56 days.

It was evident that treatment of iron deficiency anemia with BioIron™ for 56 days showed a statistically significant increase in hematologic values. Blood hemoglobin level was improved significantly ($p<0.0001$). A significant improvement in serum iron (could be correlated to the immediate release of iron from BioIron™ into the systemic circulation), total iron binding capacity and serum ferritin level was also observed (Fig. 23 and Fig. 24).

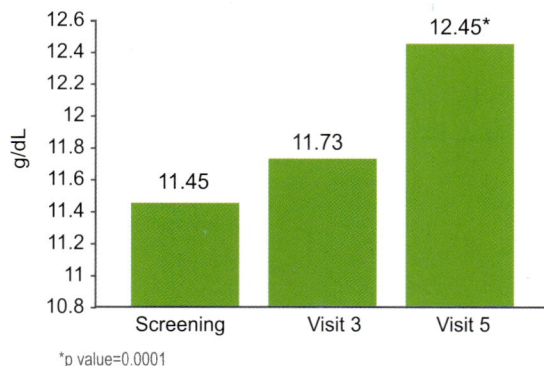

Fig. 23: Mean change in hemoglobin level over the visits.

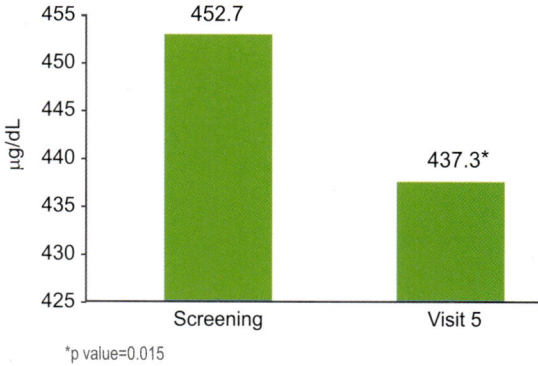

Fig. 24: Mean change in total iron binding capacity over the visits.

Thus, BioIron™ was safe and effective in the management of iron deficiency anemia without any adverse events (Majeed *et al.*, 2016b).

Piperine-associated Drug Interactions

Oral route of drug delivery is considered the most convenient and favorable mode, both in terms of therapeutic effects as well patient compliance. However, low bioavailability of a large number of synthetic compounds is the major area of concern in the modern healthcare system.

During the last couple of decades, out of several approaches that have been explored to address the issue of bioavailability, co-administration with natural compounds, as effective bioenhancers, has been of great interest.

As a result, several compounds of natural origin like piperine have been found to enhance the bioavailability of other drugs when co-administered, by various mechanisms—thus, support in exhibiting desired pharmacological effect of a drug in a most natural, safe and effective way.

Several studies have suggested that administration of piperine significantly increased the plasma concentrations of various drugs like rifampicin, phenytoin, sparteine, sulfadiazine, tetracycline, propanolol and theophylline in humans (Randhawa et al., 2011; Dudhatra et al., 2012).

The bioavailability of β-lactam antibiotics (e.g. amoxicillin trihydrate and cefotaxime sodium) was significantly enhanced with the co-administration of piperine in rats (Hiwale et al., 2002). Piperine could be used as a biological enhancer when co-administered with nimesulide in mice. In human volunteers, piperine has been reported to enhance the oral bioavailability of phenytoin, an anti-epileptic drug (Dudhatra et al., 2012).

In a randomized, placebo-controlled, 6-way, cross-over study comprising eight healthy subjects, combination of Curcumin C3 Complex® (500 mg) and BioPerine® (3 mg) or matching placebo was given orally four times over 2 days before midazolam (CYP3A probe), flurbiprofen (CYP2C9 probe) or paracetamol (dual UGT and SULT probe). Plasma and urine concentrations of drugs, metabolites and Curcumin C3 Complex® + BioPerine® at different points were measured. Results showed that there was no clinically significant effect of Curcumin C3 Complex® and BioPerine® combination on the pharmacokinetics disposition of probe drugs as compared to placebo. Thus, it was concluded that though both Curcumin C3 Complex® and BioPerine® are relatively potent inhibitors of liver enzymes involved in drug metabolism the combination does not have the ability to modify substantial disposition of medication, which are dependent on CYP3A, CYP2C9, UGT and SULT pathways—proving the safety of Curcumin C3 Complex® and BioPerine® (Volak et al., 2013).

Although a lot of research is being carried out to understand the role of piperine in enhancing the bioavailability of various formulations, especially synthetic drugs, understanding the factors that could influence the effect of piperine is of importance from biological, clinical and toxicological viewpoint. Based on recent observations from different researchers, rapid reversion of the effects of piperine with time is the reason for absence of reports on interactions of piperine with drugs in high-pepper consuming populations. Hence, it would also be important to determine the time frame for abstinence from piperine given that interethnic variability could influence pharmacokinetic profile of piperine (Han et al., 2008; Zeng et al., 2017).

These observations further implicate that time-dependent decreased impact of dietary piperine on drug pharmacokinetics underscore for the safety of piperine as well as lack of side effects on drug absorption at lower doses of piperine. It also can be emphasized that piperine is relatively a safer bioavailability enhancer with no associated drug interactions in the clinical set up (Han et al., 2008; Zeng et al., 2017).

Just to reiterate, since the content of piperine in black pepper is between 5–9%, suggesting a daily consumption of 5 mg/dose and 15 mg/day of BioPerine® may be considered safe in populations that use black pepper in their diets.

Additionally, the dose at which piperine influences bioavailability of drugs is much higher than the dose recommended for enhanced absorption of nutrients (i.e. 5 mg/dose and 15 mg/day). Hence, it would be reasonable to expect that no untoward enhanced drug absorption or pepper-associated drug interactions to occur at the dose as low as 5 mg of piperine. Moreover, taking drugs within 3–4 h of consumption of BioPerine® may be avoided as an additional precaution to avert any influence on drug-related absorption.

Overall, piperine is well known for enhancing the efficacy of pharmacologically active ingredients. Backed by several clinical trials and protected by patents, BioPerine® is a very well recognized natural bioenhancer in the market, which can be used in conjunction with several natural extracts, drugs, vitamins, minerals and antioxidants.

Chapter 4
Piperine and its Health Benefits

In the last century, although medical science was able to advance the human lifespan, its failure to tackle the problems associated with chronic disease conditions has severely blunted the impact. Hence, focus has now shifted towards alternative therapies with the evolution of integrative medicine. As a result, natural products and their derived active compounds now scientifically documented are not only medically effective in the management of various health conditions and related complications, but also cost-effective and safe.

Since time immemorial, numerous plants of high medicinal value have been effectively used to manage and prevent several diseases and associated conditions. Consequently, herbal-based ingredients or bioactives are still of significance in drug discovery. Piperine is one such phyto-ingredient among several bioactive molecules, which has been widely researched for its numerous health benefits.

This ancient spice has been documented to exhibit a wide spectrum of therapeutic potential, apart from its well known property—*bioavailability enhancement*—as an excellent adjuvant to enhance the therapeutic efficacy of the concurrently administered nutrients/drugs.

The following section details about important medicinal benefits of black pepper and/or piperine.

Antioxidant Activity

Enhanced state of oxidative stress, which is generally characterized as an imbalance between the production of reactive species and antioxidant defence activity, has been closely associated with several chronic disorders, such as cancer, diabetes, neurodegenerative and cardiovascular diseases. Various factors like exposure to air pollution, cigarette smoke, chemical and toxic fumes lead to excess of oxidative stress in the body, which in turn result in oxidation of proteins and lipids, thus affecting their structures and functions. Resultantly, reactive oxygen species (ROS) gained much attention in the last couple of decades due to their harmful action on the body (Nilani *et al.*, 2009; White *et al.*, 2014).

Several researchers have made constant efforts to assess the potent antioxidant property of natural products that represent an important source of natural antioxidants. Findings have suggested that long-term consumption of antioxidant-rich food plays a vital role in preventing or impeding the occurrence of several diseases (Singh *et al.*, 2008).

Therefore, plant-derived antioxidants are now receiving a special consideration, particularly natural products and bioactive components like piperine. These natural products are often included in the category of functional foods, in addition to providing fundamental nutritional benefits (Singh *et al.*, 2008; Butt *et al.*, 2013). According to Brewer, number of hydroxyl (-OH) groups present in the aromatic ring(s) is generally proportional to the antioxidant potential of the compound, and hence, in comparison to synthetic molecules, natural compounds would seem to have better antioxidant activity, making them appropriate ingredients of choice (Brewer, 2011).

In vitro Studies

Effect of piperine on cadmium-induced oxidative stress and immune modulation was studied in murine splenocytes. Cadmium-induced apoptosis in splenocytes was found to be preceded by increase in oxidative stress markers (i.e. ROS and GSH), decline in mitochondrial membrane potential and caspase-3 activation. Cadmium was also observed to modulate the T and B cell population, reduce blastogenesis and cytokine secretion by activated splenocytes.

Piperine treatment ameliorated the cellular events in a dose- and time-dependent manner (i.e. 1, 10 and 50 µg/ml) with 50 µg/ml dose showing complete blockade of the toxic manifestations of cadmium, with the splenocyes behaving very similar to control. Thus, it was concluded that modulation of intracellular oxidative stress signals by free radical scavenging activity and antioxidant potential of piperine could alleviate the apoptotic pathway and other cellular responses altered by cadmium treatment *in vitro* (Pathak and Khandelwal, 2007).

In vitro antioxidant activity of volatile oil and oleoresins of black pepper was carried out by Kapoor *et al*. The oleoresins extracted by both ethanol and ethyl acetate found to contain piperine as a major component (63.9 and 39.0%, respectively).

The total antioxidant activity, free radical scavenging capacity, reducing power, p-anisidine and thiobarbituric acid value of piperine was compared with synthetic antioxidants: butylated hydroxyanisole (BHA) and butylated hydroxytoluene (BHT). Both essential oils and oleoresins of piperine were found to have a stronger antioxidant activity compared to synthetic antioxidants (Kapoor *et al.*, 2009).

In a similar study, crude extracts of black pepper seeds in water and ethanol were investigated for their antioxidant and radical scavenging activities using six different assays. Results suggested that both water and ethanol extracts produced strong total antioxidant activity and peroxidation of linoleic acid emulsion inhibition was as good as standard antioxidants, such as BHA, BHT and α-tocopherol. At a concentration of 75 μg/ml water and ethanol extract showed 95.5% and 93.3% inhibition, respectively (Gülçin, 2005).

When compared with different plant extracts and phytonutrients, 98% piperine was found to have a significant nitric oxide and 2,2'-azino-bis(3-ethylbenzothiazoline-6-sulphonic acid) (ABTS) scavenging activity (Table 11). Since nitric oxide is a key mediator of inflammation, it was concluded that piperine could be used to reduce inflammation in asthma patients who are continuously under oxidative stress (Nilani et al., 2009).

Test Sample	IC_{50} value (μg/ml)	
	ABTS Method	Nitric Oxide Method
Piperine	436 ± 0.33	246 ± 0.17
Ascorbic Acid (Standard)	35 ± 0.22	30 ± 0.27
Rutin (Standard)	125 ± 0.28	185.5 ± 0.09

Table 11: Evaluation of antioxidant activity of piperine.

As oxygen radical injury and lipid peroxidation have been understood as the major causes of chronic diseases, protective effect of piperine against oxidative damage was examined by Mittal and Gupta by analyzing effect on lipid peroxidation *in vitro*. Results suggested that piperine acts as a hydroxyl radical scavenger (52% inhibition) at low concentrations (i.e. 1400 μM) with an IC_{50} of 1.23 mM, whereas it showed powerful superoxide scavenging activity with an IC_{50} of 1.82 mM. Overall, it was concluded that piperine exhibited direct antioxidant activity against various free radicals and thus proved to be a potent antioxidant against peroxide-induced tissue damage (Mittal and Gupta, 2000).

Singh *et al.* also investigated the *in vitro* antioxidant activity of different fractions (R1, R2 and R3) of black pepper fruits obtained from petroleum ether extract. The study involved elution of the fractions R1, R2 and R3 from petroleum ether and ethyl acetate in the ratio of 6:4, 5:5 and 4:6, respectively, followed by evaluation of antioxidant potential of the extract by various free radical scavenging assays.

Data from total antioxidant activity suggested that all the fractions showed concentration-dependent (50–500 µg/ml) effects, with fraction R3 producing more potent activity. The results also indicated that fractions R2 and R3 significantly inhibited ($p<0.05$) linoleic acid peroxidation (Table 12).

Concentration (µg/ml)	Inhibition (%)			
	R1	R2	R3	α-Tocopherol (Standard)
50	4.33 ± 5.25*	47.12 ± 5.24*	49.94 ± 5.78*	60.36 ± 4.35*
100	7.58 ± 2.80	50.56 ± 1.32*	52.59 ± 4.85*	65.32 ± 5.48*
250	8.18 ± 6.50	54.97 ± 2.86	56.19 ± 5.22*	68.44 ± 2.57*
500	10.21 ± 3.95	58.89 ± 2.51*	60.48 ± 3.33*	76.47 ± 5.12*

Data are mean ± SD of three measurements; *$p<0.05$ vs. Control group
R1, R2, R3: Different fractions of piperine

Table 12: Inhibition of linoleic acid peroxidation by various fractions of black pepper fruits extract.

Similar results were obtained from 2-diphenyl-1-picrylhydrazyl (DPPH) radical scavenging activity as well. The fractions R2 and R3 showed significant free radical scavenging activity ($p<0.05$) in a concentration-dependent manner (Table 13).

Concentration (µg/ml)	Inhibition (%)			
	R1	R2	R3	Butylated hydroxyanisole (BHA; Standard)
50	3.56 ± 1.32	12.58 ± 2.8*	12.32 ± 5.48*	38.59 ± 4.85*
100	5.89 ± 2.51	38.21 ± 3.95*	38.47 ± 5.12*	62.48 ± 3.33*
150	8.97 ± 2.86	43.18 ± 6.55*	43.44 ± 2.57*	70.19 ± 5.22*
200	10.12 ± 5.24	52.33 ± 5.25*	52.36 ± 4.35*	78.94 ± 5.78*
250	12.41 ± 6.62	61.24 ± 7.58	61.11 ± 4.98*	82.59 ± 4.26*

Data are mean ± SD of three measurements; *$p<0.05$ vs. Control group
R1, R2, R3: Different fractions of piperine

Table 13: DPPH free radical scavenging activity of various fractions of black pepper fruits extract.

Nitric oxide and superoxide anion radical scavenging activity results also suggested that all the fractions showed significant inhibition of nitric oxide radicals and strong superoxide radical scavenging activity, respectively. Fractions R2 and R3 reduced oxidative DNA damage in a concentration-dependent manner in hydroxyl radical scavenging activity assay.

From the study, it was apparent that petroleum ether extract of black pepper not only scavenges free radicals but inhibits the generation of free radicals as well, making it a potent antioxidant (Singh et al., 2008).

Several other *in vitro* experiments carried out by different research groups have also demonstrated the protective role of black pepper extract and/or piperine against oxidative damage and lipid peroxidation. Reddy and Lokesh reported that piperine at 600 µM has marginal inhibitory effects on ascorbate/Fe^{2+}-induced lipid peroxidation in rat liver microsomes (Reddy and Lokesh, 1992). Potent antioxidant potential of aqueous extract of black pepper as well as piperine was evaluated by Prasad *et al.* on human PMNL 5-lipoxygenase, the key enzyme involved in the biosynthesis of leukotrienes. Data showed that both black pepper extract and piperine produced a concentration-dependent inhibition of 5-lipoxygenase product 5-hydroxyeicosatetraenoic acid with IC_{50} values of 0.13 mg and 60 µM for aqueous extract of black pepper and piperine, respectively (Prasad et al., 2004). Piperine showed protection against oxidation when studied on copper ion-induced lipid peroxidation of human low-density lipoprotein (LDL). Piperine inhibited the formation of thiobarbituric acid reactive substances (TBARS) and relative electrophoretic mobility of LDL throughout the incubation period of 12 h (Naidu and Thippeswamy, 2002).

Protective effect of piperine against oxidative stress was reported in atrial myocytes (Liu et al., 2014) and copper-ascorbate-induced mitochondrial injury (Dutta et al., 2014).

In vivo Studies

Effect of piperine on chemical carcinogen-induced oxidative changes was investigated in rat intestinal model by Khajuria *et al*. Carcinogenesis was induced chemically in intestinal lumen of male rats with 7,12-dimethyl benzanthracene, dimethyl amino-methyl azobenzene and 3-methyl cholenthrene. Oxidative modifications were evaluated by determining TBARS, mainly malondialdehyde (MDA) (as a measure of lipid peroxidation), thiol status and expression of γ-glutamyl transferase and Na^+K^+ ATPase activity.

Results showed that carcinogens treatment resulted in reduction of GSH levels with substantial increase in MDA and enzyme activities. However, treatment with piperine resulted in the reversal of inhibition of MDA and other TBARS, and significantly increased the GSH levels as well as reinstated the activity of γ-glutamyl transferase and Na^+K^+ ATPase activity.

Thus, data indicated that piperine possesses a protective role against the oxidative alterations by inhibiting lipid peroxidation and mediating enhanced synthesis or transport of GSH, thereby replenishing thiol redox (Khajuria *et al.*, 1998a).

Defensive role of piperine against diabetes-induced oxidative stress was studied using 30-day streptozotocin-induced diabetic rat model. Sprague Dawley (SD) rats were treated with piperine (10 mg/kg/day; i.p.) for 14 days followed by estimation of degree of lipid peroxidation, reduced and oxidized glutathione (GSH and GSSG, respectively) content, and activities of the free radical detoxifying enzymes, such as catalase, SOD, glutathione peroxidase and glutathione reductase in tissues like liver, kidney, brain and heart.

In normal animals, piperine treatment led to 100% increase in hepatic GSSG concentration, whereas it decreased the renal GSH concentration by 35% and renal glutathione reductase activity by 25% compared to untreated controls. Piperine treatment was found to reverse the diabetic effects on GSSG concentration in brain, renal glutathione peroxidase and SOD activities, cardiac glutathione reductase activity and lipid peroxidation (Rauscher *et al.*, 2000).

The protective role of piperine in oxidative stress injuries was determined by Ma *et al*. using primary arterial cells in the oxidative injury model. The study involved isolation of primary culture of arterial muscle cells from neonatal (age: 3–5 days) New Zealand rabbits. A single cell suspension culture was prepared from isolated atria following euthanasia of rabbits. Oxidative stress in primary atrial myocytes was induced by treating with H_2O_2. Piperine group was pretreated with piperine (7×10^{-6} mol/L) for 1 h followed by 100 µmol/L H_2O_2 and cells were incubated for 2 h. Hydrogen peroxide and control groups were treated with 100 µmol/L H_2O_2 or phosphate-buffered saline for 2 h, respectively.

Various parameters analyzed were: cell viability detection, evaluation of oxidative stress markers like SOD, MDA, intracellular Ca^{2+} levels measurement and quantitative analysis of mitochondrial mRNA.

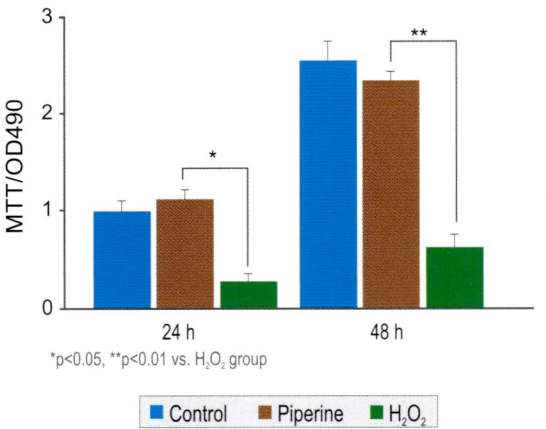

Fig. 25: Effect of piperine treatment on the cell viability.

Primary atrial myocytes from piperine-treated group showed a time-dependent significant increase in the cell viability compared to H_2O_2-treated group as observed by MTT assay (Fig. 25). These results were further corroborated with those observed with fluorescence-activated cell sorting (FACS) analysis.

Similar results were observed with SOD expression levels. Production of SOD was significantly higher in piperine-treated group ($p<0.05$), whereas significantly lower expression levels were seen in case of MDA ($p<0.01$) (Fig. 26).

Oxidative stress is known to impair the activity of ATP-dependent ion pumps in the cell membrane and in turn elevate intracellular Ca^{2+} levels. Thus, estimation of intracellular

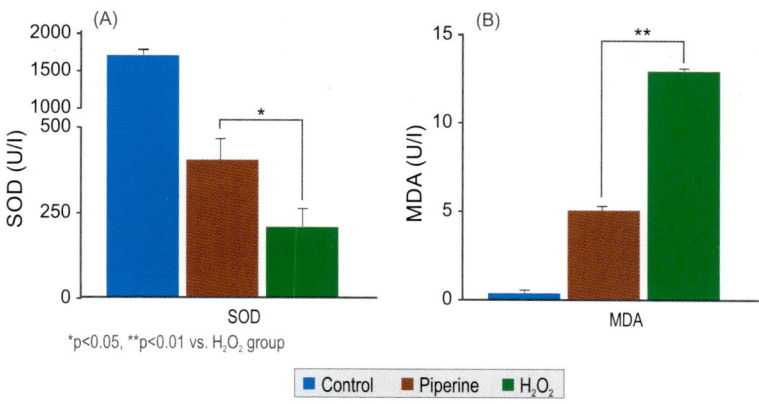

Fig. 26: Effect of piperine treatment on expression levels of (A) SOD (B) MDA.

Ca^{2+} levels revealed that piperine treatment resulted in significantly decreased Ca^{2+} levels (p<0.01) compared to H_2O_2 group. Outcome of quantitative reverse transcription polymerase chain reaction (RT-qPCR) analysis of mitochondrial mRNA expression levels in atrial myocytes showed that piperine significantly reduced the mitochondrial mRNA expression levels in a dose-dependent manner compared to H_2O_2 group.

Hence, it was concluded that piperine exhibited a protective effect against oxidative damage to primary atrial myocytes, and thus can be considered for treating oxidative stress injuries and related conditions (Ma et al., 2014).

Anti-inflammatory Activity

Inflammation is the body's attempt to protect itself from infection and forms a vital part of the body's immune response. While acute inflammation is self-resolving, chronic inflammation is associated with several adverse health conditions. Chronic inflammation is a complex biological feedback of vascular tissues to injurious stimuli, such as damaged cells, irritants or pathogens. Thus, inflammation is caused by release of chemicals from tissues and migrating cells (Bang *et al.*, 2009; Tasleem *et al.*, 2014).

Although both over-the-counter and prescription non-steroidal anti-inflammatory drugs (NSAIDs) are frequently recommended in a typical clinical practice, their use is fraught with limitations, as they are known to carry the risk of gastrointestinal toxicity upon long-term use. As a result, need for the search of compounds with no or less severe side effects has led to new interest in plant-based molecules as alternative treatments (Bang *et al.*, 2009).

Apart from culinary uses, black pepper and its major chemical constituent piperine have been demonstrated to exhibit excellent anti-inflammatory properties in various *in vitro* and *in vivo* models.

In vitro Studies

Several researchers have demonstrated potential anti-inflammatory mechanism of piperine *in vitro* in various cell types. Inhibition of LPS-induced inflammatory response by piperine was found to be via type-1 interferon mRNA expression (Bae *et al.*, 2010), extracellular signal-regulated kinases (ERK) and c-Jun N-terminal kinases (JNK) activation (Bae *et al.*, 2012), downregulating mitogen-activated protein kinase (MAPK) pathways (Hou *et al.*, 2015) and by suppressing various inflammatory mediators, such as prostaglandin E2 (PGE2), tumor necrosis factor (TNF) α, cyclooxygenase-2 (COX-2), nuclear factor kappa-B (NF-κB), matrix metalloproteinase (MMP) 3 and 13, and inducible nitric oxide synthase (iNOS) (Kim *et al.*, 2012; Ying *et al.*, 2013a; 2013b).

Effect of piperine on T lymphocyte-mediated autoimmune and chronic inflammatory disorders was studied by Doucette *et al*. It was found that piperine inhibits polyclonal and antigen-specific T lymphocyte proliferation without affecting cell viability. Additionally, piperine's ability to inhibit several key signaling pathways involved in T lymphocyte activation and the acquisition of effector function suggested that piperine might be useful in managing autoimmune conditions (Doucette *et al.*, 2015).

Recently, Rodgers *et al.* demonstrated that bone marrow-derived dendritic cells (BMDCs) that were matured in the presence of piperine (100 μM) showed reduced migration in response to CCL21 both *in vitro* and *in vivo*. Piperine treatment also impaired production of interleukin-6 (IL-6), TNF-α and monocyte chemoattractant protein-1 (MCP-1) in BMDCs stimulated with LPS. These results suggest that piperine retained dendritic cells in immature state, thus impairing their effect on activating T cells both *in vitro* and *in vivo* (Rodgers *et al.*, 2016).

In vivo Studies

Studies on chronic and acute models of inflammation in rats suggested that piperine mediated its anti-inflammatory effect by acting on early acute processes and chronic granulative changes, as well as partially through pituitary-adrenal axis stimulation (Mujumdar *et al.*, 1990). Piperine was also thought to elucidate its anti-inflammatory activity by inhibiting nitric oxide and TNF-α production both *in vitro* and *in vivo* (Pradeep and Kuttan, 2003).

Immuno-modulatory and anti-inflammatory response of piperine was evaluated by Aswar *et al.* in ovalbumin-induced paw edema model. In this study, animals were treated with different doses of piperine (i.e. 10, 20 and 40 mg/kg; p.o.) or cetrizine (10 mg/kg; p.o.) for 4 days. On day 4, all mice except normal control were challenged with sensitization solution having ovalbumin (10 μg/0.1 ml) by sub-plantar administration in the hind paw. Inhibition of paw edema was measured post 1, 3 and 24 h of ovalbumin sensitization using the pathysmometer. A significant reduction in paw thickness ($p<0.001$) was seen in piperine-treated animals at 1 h time point. Furthermore, mast cell degranulation data also showed that at 20 and 40 mg/kg piperine possesses mast cell-stabilizing activity, thereby inhibiting the release of pro-inflammatory mediators like histamine, IL-6, IL-1β and immunoglobulin E (IgE) (Aswar *et al.*, 2015).

In experimental periodontitis model, piperine evidently exhibited protective role against inflammation, alveolar bone loss and collagen fibre degradation in a dose-dependent manner. Piperine inhibited alveolar bone loss as well as reformed trabecula microstructures. Soft tissue histopathology demonstrated that piperine reduced the infiltration of inflammatory cells and limited the fractions of degraded areas in collagen fibers at 50 and 100 mg/kg dose. Expression of IL-1β, MMP-8 and MMP-13 was downregulated at 100 mg/kg concentration. Overall, it was concluded that efficacy of piperine may be attributed to its inhibitory action on the expression of these pro-inflammatory markers (Dong *et al.*, 2015).

The anti-inflammatory activity of crude extracts of black pepper and isolated pure piperine were compared in carrageenan-induced paw edema in rats by Tasleem *et al*. Animals were injected with carrageenan in left hind paw post 1 h of oral administration of diclofenac (a standard drug), test compounds or saline water (control). Pure piperine showed a dose-dependent inhibition of edema compared to control with maximum inhibition at 15 mg/kg after 2 h. Crude extracts of black pepper (i.e. hexane and ethanol extracts) showed maximum activity at 10 mg/kg after 1 h compared to control. Acute toxicity study of black pepper extract revealed no mortality at 15 mg/kg dose. Thus, the study concluded that piperine and crude extracts of black pepper possessed potent anti-inflammatory activity in rodents (Tasleem *et al.*, 2014).

Recently, Zhai *et al*. explored the possible mechanism of action and anti-inflammatory effect of piperine on *Staphylococcus aureus* endometritis in mice model. In this study, 60 female BALB/c mice were infected with *S. aureus* in the uterus followed by intraperitoneal injection of piperine (three times every 6 h) 24 h after *S. aureus* infection. Mice were equally divided into control healthy mice, *S. aureus*-infected mice without any treatment, piperine-treated mice at three different concentrations (25, 50 or 100 mg/kg) and dexamethasone (DEX) treatment. The uterine tissues were analyzed for histopathological changes, cytokines expression (i.e. TNF-α, IL-1β, IL-6 and IL-10) using enzyme-linked immunosorbent assay (ELISA) and qPCR methods, expression of toll-like receptors (TLR-2 and TLR-4), NF-κB and MAPK signaling pathways using Western blot assays.

Results from histopathological analysis revealed that *S. aureus* treatment produced inflammatory injury with destruction of epithelial cells and infiltration of uterine tissues with neutrophils and macrophages, which was ameliorated by piperine treatment in a dose-dependent manner. Expression of pro-inflammatory cytokines like TNF-α, IL-1β and IL-6 was increased in *S. aureus*-treated group, whereas piperine treatment reversed these effects as well as improved the expression of IL-10, an anti-inflammatory cytokine, in a dose-dependent way. Furthermore, respective mRNA expression was consistent with the protein expression. Similar results were observed with mRNA levels of TLR-2 and TLR-4 (Fig. 27). Piperine treatment also resulted in significant inhibition of both NF-κB and MAPK pathways (Fig. 28), which are known to play a major role in the inflammatory reaction and development of endometrial inflammation, respectively.

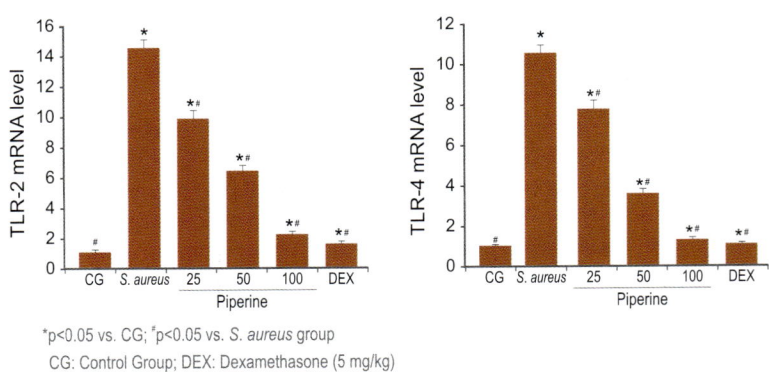

*p<0.05 vs. CG; #p<0.05 vs. *S. aureus* group
CG: Control Group; DEX: Dexamethasone (5 mg/kg)

Fig. 27: Effect of piperine on mRNA expression levels of TLR-2 and TLR-4.

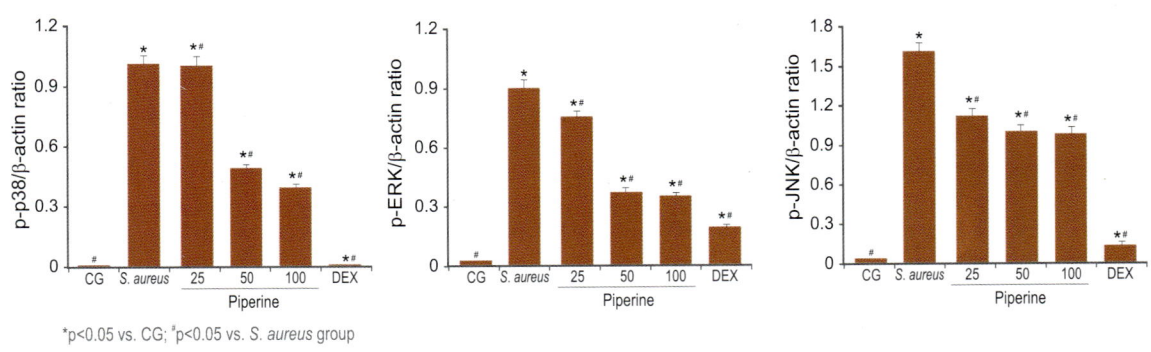

*p<0.05 vs. CG; #p<0.05 vs. *S. aureus* group
CG: Control Group; DEX: Dexamethasone (5 mg/kg)

Fig. 28: Effect of piperine on activation of MAPK pathways.

In conclusion, piperine may be useful against *S. aureus*-induced endometritis and other infections due to its potential anti-inflammatory actions (Zhai et al., 2016).

Several researchers demonstrated protective role of piperine in a variety of inflammatory conditions, such as LPS-induced acute lung injury (Lu et al., 2016), cerulein-induced acute pancreatitis (Bae et al., 2011) and streptozotocin-induced diabetic nephropathy focusing on inflammation (Samra et al., 2016). The anti-inflammatory effect of piperine was mediated by inhibiting activation of NF-κB, MAPK, NLRP3 and other pro-inflammatory pathways.

Therapeutic role of piperine was also evident from various animal models for irritable bowel disease, wherein piperine prevented or reduced the inflammation at colorectal sites by downregulating TLR-4 pathway and other inflammatory mediators (Gupta et al., 2015), and by acting as a potential agonist and inducer of PXR, thus inducing CYP3A4 gene expression at mRNA and protein levels (Hu et al., 2015).

Furthermore, piperine was found to be safe and effective therapy for rheumatoid arthritis in different animal models like collagen- (Umar et al., 2013) and adjuvant-induced arthritis (Murunikkara et al., 2012), as well as monosodium urate crystal-induced model of gouty arthritis (Sabina et al., 2011). Overall, these studies clearly indicate that piperine could be a potent anti-inflammatory agent because of its ability to alter a number of factors known to be involved in inflammatory conditions.

Li *et al.* carried out *in vitro* and *ex vivo* experiments to study anti-inflammatory and anti-catabolic effects of piperine in preventing the breakdown of intervertebral disc (IVD) in rats using LPS-induced inflammation in rat nucleus pulposus cells culture and IVD organ culture models. Intervertebral disc degeneration (IDD) is a degenerative disease, wherein, the extracellular matrix in IVD is lost due to the activity of MMPs.

The nucleus pulposus cells were isolated from lumbar spines of SD rats using standard enzymatic digestion and were incubated with piperine (0–100 mg/ml) for 2 h, followed by LPS stimulation (10 μg/ml) for 24 h. Similarly, organ culture was prepared by isolating the motion segment from each lumbar vertebrae (including upper and lower end plate, and whole disc) and was maintained for 14 days with or without LPS and different concentrations of piperine. Various parameters like cell viability, proteoglycan content, RT-PCR and ELISA for mRNA and protein level of various matrix-degrading enzymes like MMP-3 and MMP-13, a disintegrin and metalloproteinase with thrombospondin motifs (ADAMTS-4 and ADAMTS-5), and several genes of inflammatory factors, and histological analysis of discs were evaluated.

Chapter 4
PIPERINE AND ITS HEALTH BENEFITS

Data from cell viability assay revealed no cytotoxicity from piperine at tested concentrations (i.e. 100–200 μg/ml). Piperine was found to inhibit LPS-induced expression and production of inflammatory factors and catabolic proteases in nucleus pulposus cells culture model in a dose-dependent manner. Both ELISA and RT-PCR data showed that piperine significantly inhibited LPS-induced secretion of MMP-3 and MMP-13, and downregulated mRNA expression levels of ADAMTS-4, ADAMTS-5, MMP-3 and MMP-13, respectively (Fig. 29).

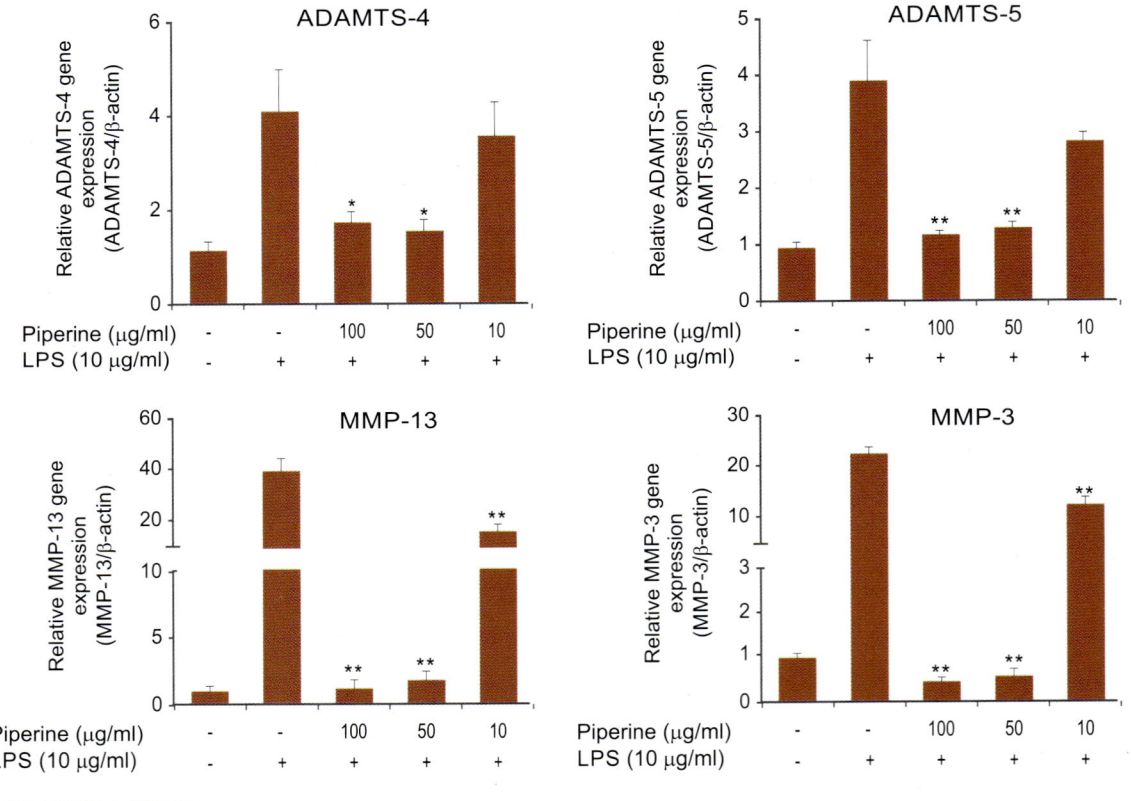

*p<0.05, **p<0.01 vs. LPS group

Fig. 29: Effect of piperine on gene expression of MMPs and ADAMTS (RT-PCR analysis).

Western blot analysis showed potential involvement of the signal transduction pathways and mechanism of anti-inflammatory action of piperine. Results demonstrated that LPS significantly induced the activation of MAPKs and NF-κB, which were dose-dependently inhibited by piperine.

Piperine also demonstrated inhibition of gene expression of inflammatory cytokines (IL-1β, TNF-α and IL-6), aggrecan, collagen-II, iNOS and nitric oxide production. Furthermore, immunohistochemical quantification of collagen-II revealed that piperine significantly attenuated (p<0.01) the LPS-induced collagen loss, especially on day 7 (Fig. 30).

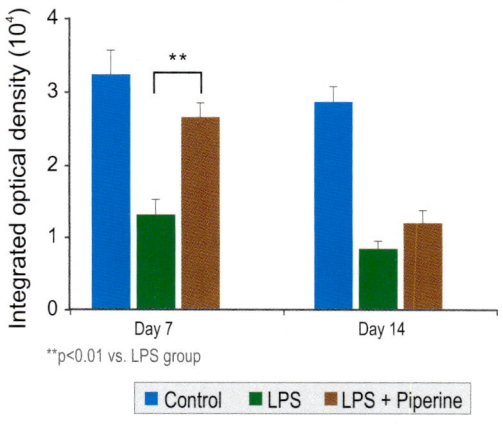

Fig. 30: Effect of piperine treatment on collagen-II loss.

Histopathological analysis also demonstrated that piperine significantly reduced the IVD degeneration in organ culture model at 100 μg/ml concentration.

Overall, these results suggested that piperine significantly antagonized LPS-mediated inflammatory pathways in both nucleus pulposus cells and organ culture models, supporting its potential anti-inflammatory role in the treatment of disc degenerative disorders (Li et al., 2015b).

In another study, anti-inflammatory, nociceptive and anti-arthritic activity of piperine was determined by Bang et al. In vitro analysis involved testing of anti-inflammatory activity in IL-1β-stimulated fibroblast-like synoviocytes (FLS), derived from rheumatoid arthritis patients, whereas nociceptive and anti-arthritic efficacy tests were carried out in rat models of carrageenan-induced acute paw pain and arthritis, respectively.

Synovial tissues were collected from arthritic patients who underwent therapeutic joint surgery to isolate FLS and were subjected to semiquantitative RT-PCR, ELISA and Western blot analysis, following treatment with different concentrations of piperine. In animal model, SD rats were given the intraplantar injection of 0.1 ml carrageenan (1%) in the posterior right paw to induce hyperalgesia. Rats were divided into different groups and treated with piperine (20 and 100 mg/kg), celecoxib (100 mg/kg) or no treatment. Similarly, in carrageenan-induced arthritic rat model, arthritic inflammation was induced by a single injection of 3% carrageenan into left tibiotarsal ankle joint. Arthritic progression was evaluated every day up to day 9 using different parameters like paw volume, squeaking score in the ankle flexion test and weight distribution ratio, which are considered as behavioral indicators of carrageenan-induced arthritis.

The *in vitro* anti-inflammatory efficacy results showed that IL-1β treatment induced the production of IL-6 and PGE2, which were significantly inhibited by piperine in a dose-dependent manner. Both protein and mRNA expression levels of IL-6 and COX-2 were inhibited upon piperine treatment. Additionally, piperine treatment resulted in inhibition of MMP-13 expression at both protein and mRNA levels, and was thought to act via inhibition of ERK1/2 signaling pathway by blocking the migration of activator protein 1 (AP-1) into the nucleus.

Piperine at 100 mg/kg dose demonstrated anti-nociceptive effects in a rat model of carrageenan-induced paw hyperalgesia. In the arthritis model, at 100 mg/kg dose, piperine produced a significant reduction in paw volume ($p<0.05$) compared to control group and showed almost the same efficacy as prednisolone, a standard drug (Fig. 31A). Squeaking score, which was based on the number of vocalizations caused by flexion or extension of the inflamed ankle, was found to be started decreasing from day 5 onwards in piperine group (100 mg/kg) through day 9 (Fig. 31B).

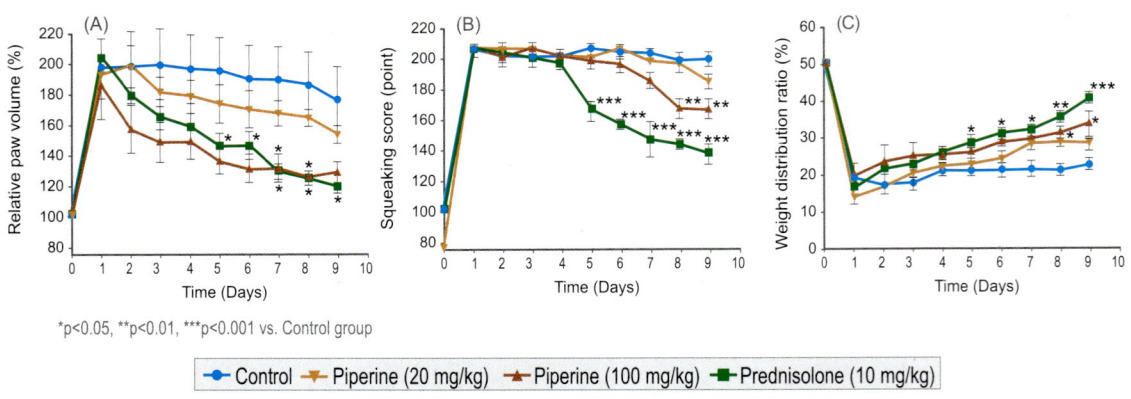

Fig. 31: Anti-arthritic effect of piperine in carrageenan-induced arthritic rat model.

Chapter 4
PIPERINE AND ITS HEALTH BENEFITS

Similarly, data from weight distribution ratio suggested that group receiving 100 mg/kg dose of piperine resulted in significant recovery on days 8 and 9 ($p<0.05$) (Fig. 31C).

The degree of inflammation was diminished in group treated with 100 mg/kg piperine indicating anti-inflammatory action, as observed by the histopathological evaluation of ankle joints. Thus, it was concluded that piperine demonstrated anti-inflammatory, nociceptive and anti-arthritic activities, and hence should be further studied for its potential as a dietary supplement or therapeutic drug (Bang *et al.*, 2009).

Recently, role of piperine in improving symptoms related to nephrotic syndrome were well established *in vivo* by Kakalij *et al.* It was postulated that protective role of piperine could be due to its immunomodulatory and anti-inflammatory potential (Kakalij *et al.*, 2016).

In vivo anti-inflammatory and anti-arthritic activities of combination of *trans*-cinnamaldehyde, an essential oil present in the bark of cinnamon (Williams *et al.*, 2015; Chen *et al.*, 2016), and piperine were studied by Jadhav and Prabhavalkar, using rat models of carrageenan-induced paw edema and complete Freund's adjuvant (CFA) induced arthritis, respectively.

In carrageenan model, male SD rats were treated with piperine (15 mg/kg), *trans*-cinnamaldehyde (5 mg/kg) or the combination of piperine (8 mg/kg) and *trans*-cinnamaldehyde (5 mg/kg) followed by carrageeenan (1%) administration in the hind paw 30 min. post drugs treatment. Paw edema was measured at different time points up to 4 h using plethysmometer. In CFA model, arthritis was induced by CFA followed by subsequent treatment (same as above).

A significant reduction in the paw edema was observed in all treatment groups in carrageenan model from the first hour through fourth when compared to control group. At 4 h time point, anti-inflammatory activity of the combination treatment was comparable with that of indomethacin (3 mg/kg), a standard drug. Similarly, in CFA model, the combination group showed significantly reduced swelling in the CFA-injected paws, inhibition of inflammatory response in non-injected sites and inhibition of T-cells activation and proliferation, thereby inhibiting the secondary lesions. Data from the histopathological examination also validated the anti-arthritic effect of the combination.

Hence, it was concluded that piperine alone as well as in combination with *trans*-cinnamaldehyde was beneficial in alleviating inflammatory responses in animal models for inflammation and arthritis (Jadhav and Prabhavalkar, 2015; 2016).

Anticancer Activity

Across the world, cancer is being considered as one of the highest impacting diseases with significant morbidity and mortality rates. Though current therapeutic options, such as radiotherapy and chemotherapy are benefiting cancer patients in terms of their health re-establishment, the treatment is very painful and patients' immunological system is severely compromised as these procedures are not cell-selective. Additionally, treatment cost is very high and also with myriad side effects (Paarakh et al., 2015).

Since ancient times, spices have not only been used as preservatives but also as traditional medicines—owing to the rich source of phytoactives—in managing the risk of chronic diseases like cancer and related complications. As a result, recent developments in the field of anticancer therapy have focused on novel strategies involving plant-based approach to treat malignancy or chemoprevention. One such plant is *Piper nigrum* (Butt et al., 2013; Paarakh et al., 2015).

Extensive research has been carried out to explore the chemopreventive effects, cytotoxic activity and possible mechanism of action of black pepper and piperine against various cancer types, including pancreatic, colon, prostate, breast and lung cancer both *in vitro* and *in vivo*.

In vitro Studies

A number of studies have shown the relationship between ROS-dependent cell cycle arrest and apoptosis induced by *Piper nigrum* and piperine, and their cytotoxic/apoptotic/antitumor activity. Recently, both piperine and ethanolic extract of *Piper nigrum* have been shown to exhibit cytotoxic and antiproliferative effect via ROS overproduction, which in turn results in oxidative stress, leading to cell cycle arrest at G_1/S phase and apoptosis in HT-29 and MCF-7 cells, respectively (Yaffe *et al.*, 2015; de Souza Grinevicius *et al.*, 2016). Similar results were seen when effect of piperine on the growth of HRT-18 human rectal adenocarcinoma cells was studied. Flow cytometric analysis data revealed that piperine inhibited cell cycle progression—suggesting cytostatic and/or cytotoxic effect (Yaffe *et al.*, 2013).

Both *Piper nigrum* extract and piperine were found to exhibit inhibitory effects on TNF-induced NF-κB activation, human tumor cell proliferation, COX enzymes and lipid peroxidation (Liu *et al.*, 2010). Piperine was also found to exert the cytotoxic effect against human lung cancer A549 cells by causing cell DNA damage, cell cycle arrest at G_2/M phase and activating caspase-3 and caspase-9 cascades in cells, resulting in apoptosis as well as increased Bax/Bcl-2 ratio (Lin *et al.*, 2014). Anticancer effects of piperine were thought to be produced by regulating IL-6 expression through the suppression of p38 MAPK and signal transducer and activator of transcription 3 (STAT3) (Xia *et al.*, 2015) and anti-proliferative effects by inducing cell cycle arrest and autophagy in human prostate cancer cells (Ouyang *et al.*, 2013).

Results from another study showed that piperine re-sensitizes P-gp, multidrug resistance protein 1 (MRP1) and breast cancer resistance protein-dependent multidrug resistant cancer cells (Li *et al.*, 2011). Further studies have also demonstrated that piperine's antitumor activity is because of its influence in various pathways, including ERK1/2, p38 MAPK, c-JNK, c-Fos, nuclear factor of activated T-cells cytoplasmic 1 and Akt signaling pathways (Reen *et al.*, 1996; Pradeep and Kuttan, 2004; Do *et al.*, 2013; Deepak *et al.*, 2015; Zhang *et al.*, 2015).

Radiosensitizers have been used to augment the effect of ionizing radiation in treating various cancer forms in human. Tak *et al.* evaluated the radiosensitizing effects of resveratrol and piperine on cancer cells. During the study, cancer cell lines when treated with resveratrol and piperine produced significantly augmented apoptosis induced by ionizing radiation as well as loss of mitochondrial membrane potential suggesting ROS overproduction. Hence, it was concluded that natural products like resveratrol and piperine as sensitizers can offer promising therapeutic adjunct in treating cancer in human (Tak et al., 2012).

In another study, treatment with ethanolic extract of black pepper resulted in DNA damage and decreased cell viability in MCF-7 and HT-29 cells (EC_{50}=27.1 ± 2.0 and 80.5 ± 6.6 µg/ml, respectively). Additionally, expression of Bax and p53 was enhanced, whereas that of Bcl-xL and cyclin A was decreased upon treatment with the extract. Enhanced activity of glutathione reductase, SOD and catalase, and decreased GSH concentration was observed in black pepper extract-treated tumor tissues. Thus, researchers concluded that ethanolic extract of black pepper has cytotoxic and anti-proliferative effect on cancer cell lines (de Souza Grinevicius et al., 2016).

Similarly, Fofaria *et al.* demonstrated anti-proliferative effect of piperine in murine and human melanoma cells. B16 F0 cells from C57Bl/6 mice and SK MEL 28 and A375 cells, obtained from a human male subject were used for the study. This *in vitro* study involved various assays to determine cell survival, cell cycle analysis, apoptosis and ROS generation.

Treatment with varying concentration of piperine (75–300 µM) resulted in a significant reduction of cell survival across all the cell lines at 24, 48 and 72 h time points. Higher concentration of piperine (300 µM) was found to suppress the growth of B16 F0 cells almost completely, whereas SK MEL 28 and A375 cells were inhibited by 90% at 48 and 72 h. Cell cycle analysis also revealed that piperine at 150 µM resulted in significant accumulation of B16 F0 and SK MEL 28 cells in G_1 phase with a concomitant decrease of the cells in S and G_2/M phase was seen when treated with piperine at varying concentrations (100–200 µM) (Fig. 32).

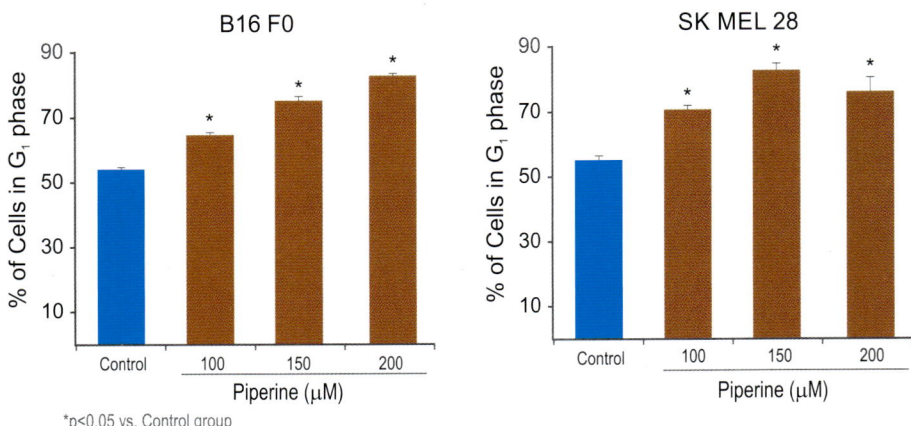

Fig. 32: Concentration-dependent effect of piperine on number of melanoma cells in G_1 phase.

This observation was further validated when piperine treatment resulted in significant phosphorylation of H2A.X, a marker of DNA damage, in a concentration-dependent manner in both the cell lines. Additionally, a drastic reduction in the expression of DNA polymerase β, an enzyme responsible for the repair of DNA strand damage, was witnessed upon piperine treatment.

The molecular mechanism behind the cell cycle arrest of melanoma cells in G_1 phase was further corroborated when results proved the involvement of regulatory proteins like ATR, Chk1, p53 and p21.

Data from the apoptosis assay revealed that varying concentrations of piperine induced significant apoptosis in both the cell lines, with B16 F0 being more sensitive than SK MEL 28 cells (i.e. 60% vs. 45% at 200 μM) (Fig. 33). In addition, downregulation of key proteins, such as XIAP, an inhibitor of apoptosis, and Bid (full length) confirmed by Western blot analysis further validated the role of piperine in mitochondrial death pathway.

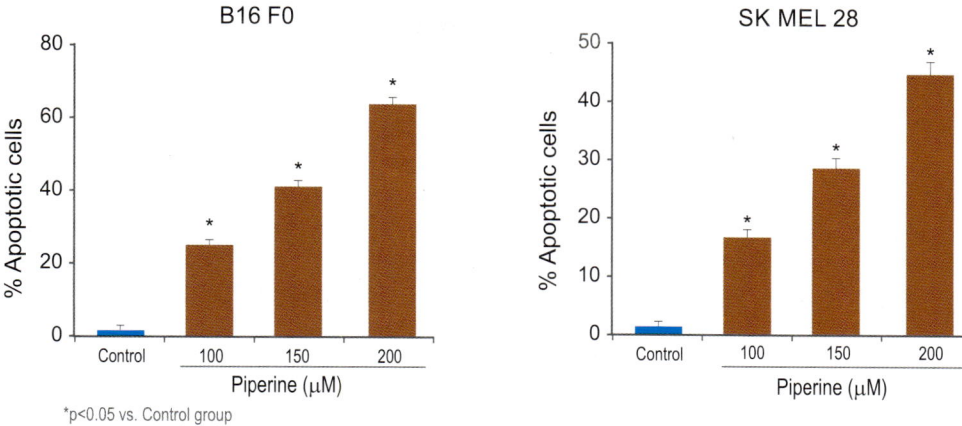

Fig. 33: Concentration-dependent effect of piperine on percentage of apoptotic cells in different types of melanoma cells.

Furthermore, piperine treatment caused early and persistent generation of ROS in both the cells in a time- and concentration-dependent manner. Taken together, results suggested that piperine-mediated ROS generation plays a critical role in inducing DNA damage leading to G_1 cell cycle arrest and apoptosis in melanoma cells (Fofaria et al., 2014).

Inhibitory effect of piperine on the growth and adhesion of *Helicobacter pylori* to gastric adenocarcinoma cells was investigated by Tharmalingam *et al*. In this study, piperine demonstrated significant growth inhibitory activity against different strains of *H. pylori* (Fig. 34) with IC_{50} of 115 µM against *H. pylori* strain 60190.

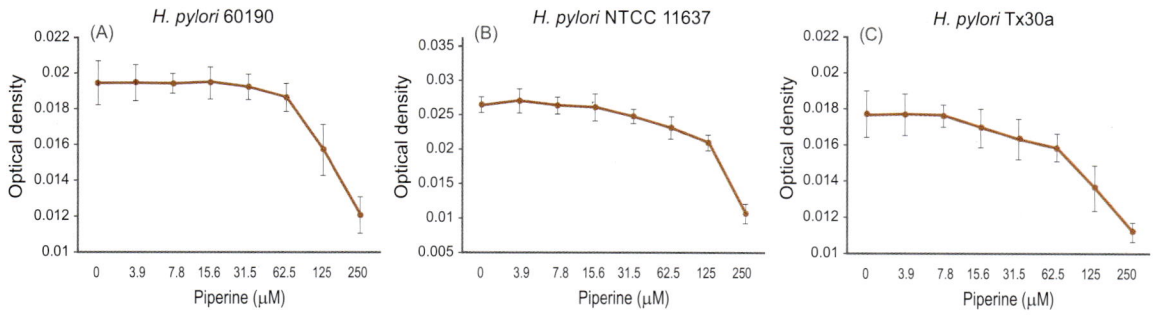

Fig. 34: Growth inhibitory activity of piperine on different strains of *Helicobacter pylori*.

Piperine treatment at different concentrations (50–125 µM) during the infective stage produced concentration-dependent inhibition of *H. pylori* strain 60190 adhesion to gastric epithelial cells (Fig. 35A). In a similar assay, effect of piperine (100 µM) on bacterial adhesion to adenocarcinoma cells was studied at higher multiplicity of infection during infection and pretreatment. It was observed that piperine treatment significantly reduced the bacterial adhesion to adenocarcinoma cells, during infection ($p<0.01$) as well as bacteria pretreatment ($p<0.05$) by 40% and 25%, respectively at higher multiplicity of infection of 100 and 200 (Fig. 35B).

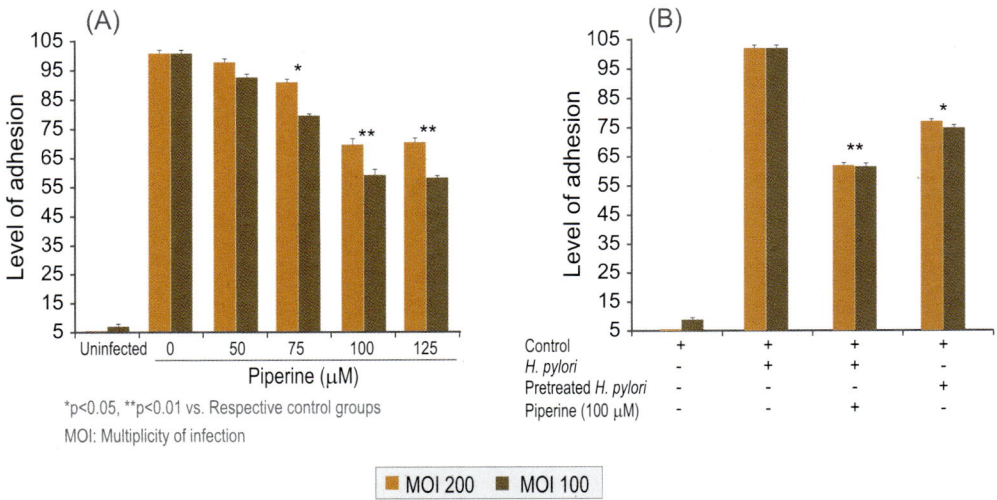

Fig. 35: Adhesion inhibitory activity of piperine on *H. pylori* in (A) Gastric adenocarcinoma cells (B) Effect of piperine during infection and pretreatment.

Additionally, piperine treatment also abated the motility of *H. pylori* in a concentration-dependent manner (50–125 µM). The expression of flagellar integral membrane protein and the flagellar hook component were significantly reduced in piperine-treated bacteria, suggesting that piperine-induced inhibition of adhesion was due to decreased motility—resulting in lower attraction and adhesion to gastric epithelial cells. In summary, piperine effectively inhibited the growth and adhesion of *H. pylori* bacteria to adenocarcinoma cells (Tharmalingam et al., 2014).

Based on this report (Tharmalingam *et al.*, 2014) another *in vitro* study was carried out by the same group to determine the role of piperine in treating *H. pylori* infection. Results suggested that piperine produced cytotoxic effects against adenocarcinoma cells at concentration of 100 μM or more. Treatment with piperine resulted in diminished E-cadherin cleavage as well as reduced β-catenin expression compared to untreated *H. pylori*-infected cells. Piperine also suppressed IL-8 mRNA expression and IL-8 protein synthesis at different time points in *H. pylori*-infected host cells. Overall, it was concluded that piperine's protection against *H. pylori* infection in adenocarcinoma cells could be due to reduced toxin secretion and toxin entry as described previously, along with reduced E-cadherin cleavage, level of β-catenin and IL-8-mediated inflammation (Tharmalingam *et al.*, 2016).

A couple of other studies have also highlighted the potential role of piperine as a cytotoxic and anti-angiogenic agent. In one study, the MTT assay demonstrated that piperine has cytotoxic effect against HeLa cells with IC_{50} value of 61.94 ± 0.054 μg/ml (Paarakh *et al.*, 2015). In another study, effect of piperine on angiogenesis in human umbilical vein endothelial cells was investigated by Doucette *et al*. Piperine was found to inhibit multiple aspects of angiogenic process by inhibiting the phosphoinositide-3 kinase/Akt signaling cascade, which plays an important role in angiogenesis (Doucette *et al.*, 2013).

In vivo Studies

The potential of piperine as cytoprotective and chemopreventive agent against benzo(a)pyrene (BAP) induced experimental lung carcinogenesis has been vastly investigated by Selvendiran *et al*. Based on several experiments carried out by the group, it can be inferred that piperine extends its chemopreventive effect by modulating lipid peroxidation and augmenting antioxidant defence mechanism (Selvendiran *et al*., 2003; 2004a; 2005a), wherein oral administration of piperine effectively suppressed BAP-induced lung carcinogenesis by reducing the extent of lipid peroxidation with concomitant increase in enzymatic and non-enzymatic antioxidant activities.

Similar results were obtained when role of oral supplementation of piperine was evaluated in experimental lung carcinogenesis initiated by BAP and buccal pouch carcinogenesis induced by 7,12-dimethyl benz(a)anthracene. Enhanced ATPase enzymes activity in erythrocyte membrane and tissues were reversed to normal range by piperine treatment—suggesting that the primarily beneficial effects of piperine is exerted during initiation phase and post-initiation stage of the carcinogenesis (Selvendiran and Sakthisekaran, 2004). Piperine also reduced the DNA damage and DNA-protein cross links (Selvendiran *et al*., 2005b), and modulated the biochemical changes at molecular level (Krishnakumar *et al*., 2009).

Furthermore, administration of piperine significantly decreased the levels of total protein and protein-bound carbonyls, nucleic acid content and polyamine synthesis, thus offering protection from protein damage and also controlling cell proliferation (Selvendiran *et al*., 2004b; 2006).

Anti-metastatic activity of piperine against B16F-10 melanoma cells-induced lung metastasis in C57Bl/6 mice revealed significant reduction in tumor nodule formation (95.2%), lung collagen hydroxyproline levels (2.59 µg/mg vs. 22.37 µg/mg protein) in piperine-treated animals compared to metastatized lung samples. Histopathology of the lung tissues also correlated with the lifespan of piperine-treated animals, wherein mice were found to survive the experimental duration (i.e. 90 days) (Pradeep and Kuttan, 2002).

In a murine breast cancer model, effects of piperine on the tumor growth and metastasis of 4T1 breast cancer were evaluated *in vitro* and *in vivo* by Lai *et al*. Piperine produced a time- and dose-dependent (35–280 µmol/L) inhibition of growth of 4T1 mammary carcinoma cells (Fig. 36A) with IC_{50} values 105 ± 1.08 and 78.52 ± 1.06 µmol/L at 48 and 72 h, respectively. Treatment of 4T1 cells with piperine (70–280 µmol/L) induced the apoptosis in a concentration-dependent manner, which was accompanied by upregulation of caspase-3 (Fig. 36B).

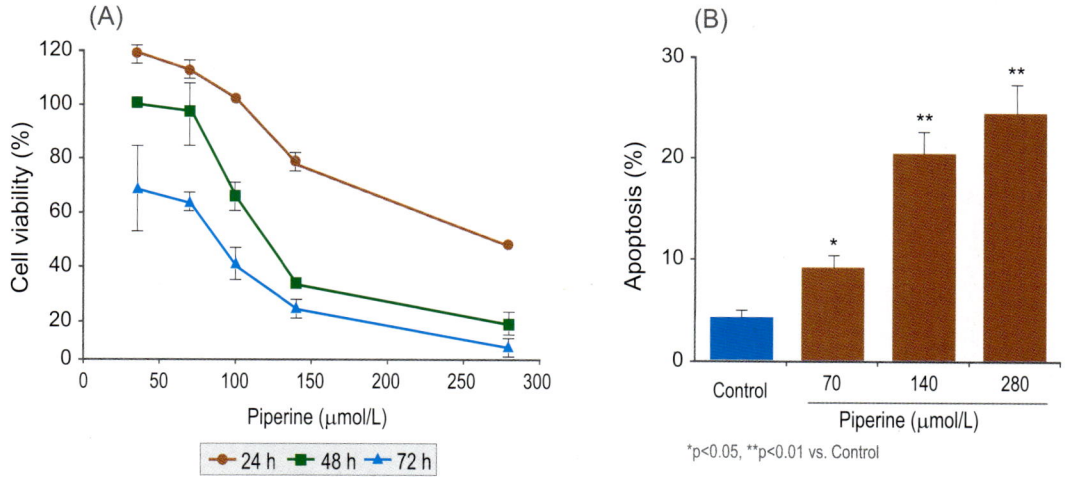

Fig. 36: Effect of piperine treatment on (A) Cell viability (B) Apoptosis in 4T1 cells.

Piperine treatment (140 and 280 µmol/L) also led to significant increase in the percentage of cells in G_2/M phase along with downregulation of the expression of cyclin B1. Piperine was found to inhibit the migration of 4T1 cells *in vitro* in a concentration-dependent manner. Furthermore, concentration-dependent decrease in the mRNA expression of MMP-9 and MMP-13 in 4T1 cells was observed when treated with piperine.

In vivo antitumor activity of piperine was evaluated in mice mammary carcinoma model. In this test, female BALB/c mice syngenic to 4T1 cells were inoculated subcutaneously with 5×10^5 4T1 cells. Post 3 days of implantation, piperine (2.5 and 5 mg/kg) was administered into the tumors every three days for three times. A dose-dependent inhibition of tumor growth (Fig. 37A) along with increased levels of caspase-3 and reduced cyclin B1 was observed in piperine-treated animals—advocating the role of piperine in regulating apoptotic proteins and cell cycle-related regulatory proteins. Histological examination of tumor tissues collected on day 20 showed that tumors excised from the mice treated with piperine exhibited wide areas of coagulative necrosis. Examination of lung samples collected on day 30 post-inoculation also revealed that piperine at 5 mg/kg significantly inhibited lung metastasis (Fig. 37B)—thus, implicating that piperine not only suppressed the local primary tumor growth, but also successfully regulated the rate of spontaneous metastasis.

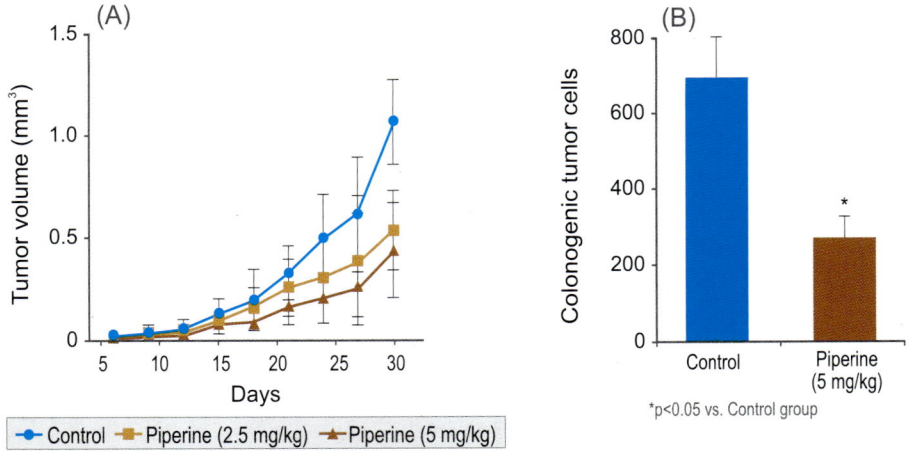

Fig. 37: Effect of piperine treatment on (A) Tumor growth (B) Lung metastasis in 4T1 inoculated cells.

Authors concluded that piperine effectively inhibited tumor growth and metastasis by inhibiting cell viability, and inducing cell apoptosis and cell cycle blockage both *in vitro* and *in vivo*. Hence, it could be a useful adjunct in cancer therapy (Lai et al., 2012).

In another study, it was observed that anti-mutagenic potential of piperine could be due to its influence on chromosomal aberrations. Chromosomal analysis of bone marrow samples from male Wistar rats treated with piperine (100–800 mg/kg), followed by challenge with cyclophosphamide (50 mg/kg) showed that at 100 mg/kg piperine significantly decreased the chromosomal aberrations (Wongpa et al., 2007).

Beneficial role of piperine in enhancing the efficacy of TNF-related apoptosis-inducing ligand (TRAIL) based therapies in triple-negative breast cancer (TNBC) cells was studied *in vitro* and *in vivo*. Piperine was found to induce sensitivity to TRAIL through suppression of surviving expression and p65 phosphorylation (Abdelhamed et al., 2014). In a similar study, piperine inhibited *in vitro* growth of TNBC cells without affecting normal mammary epithelial cell growth by decreasing the percentage of TNBC cells in the G_2 phase, cell cycle-associated protein expression and increased expression of p21 (Waf1/Cip1). Additionally, combined treatment with piperine and γ-radiation was found to be more cytotoxic for TNBC cells than γ-radiation alone. Growth of TNBC xenografts in immune-deficient mice was also inhibited by piperine upon intra-tumoral administration (Greenshields et al., 2015).

Based on the reported studies that suggested inhibitory activity of piperine against CYP3A4, a drug-metabolizing enzyme, a study was planned by Makhov *et al.* to investigate pharmacokinetic and anticancer effects of piperine when combined with docetaxel in a xenograft animal model of human prostate cancer.

The effect of piperine on hepatic activity of CYP3A4 was studied by administering 50 mg/kg/dose piperine orally to C.B17/Icr-scid mice. Post 1 h of treatment, animals were euthanized and liver homogenates from control and treatment animals were collected to measure the activity of CYP3A4. Similarly, pharmacokinetic study was carried out to investigate the effect of piperine-mediated CYP3A4 inhibition on pharmacokinetics of docetaxel. Here, C.B17/Icr-scid mice were administered piperine (100 mg/kg; p.o.) followed by docetaxel (12.5 mg/kg; i.v.). Blood samples were collected to measure the plasma concentration of docetaxel alone or in combination with piperine.

To understand the synergestic effect of piperine and docetaxel in anticancer activity, 6-week-old C.B17/Icr-scid mice were inoculated with castration-resistant PC-3 xenograft tumors (1×10^6). Two weeks after the tumor implantation, animals were randomly divided into four groups and were treated with piperine (100 mg/kg/dose; p.o., weekly), docetaxel (12.5 mg/kg/dose; i.v., weekly), piperine-docetaxel combination or no treatment. Piperine was administered 1 h prior to the docetaxel injection.

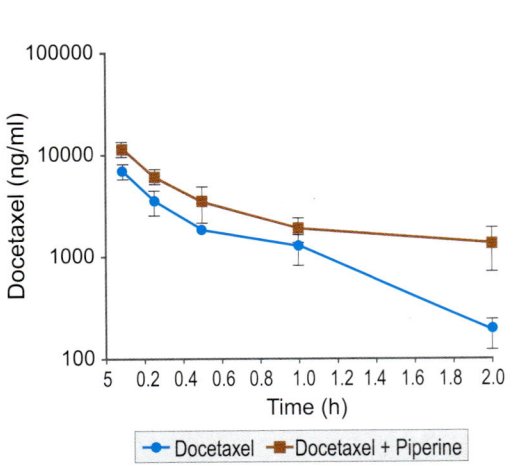

Fig. 38: Effect of co-administration of piperine on the plasma levels of docetaxel.

Hepatic cells isolated from piperine-treated mice significantly reduced the CYP3A4 activity compared to control samples, confirming CYP3A4 inhibitory activity of piperine. Likewise, administration of piperine resulted in prolonged plasma levels of docetaxel in comparison to docetaxel alone group in a time-dependent manner, particularly between 1 h and 2 h post docetaxel injection (i.e. 7-fold increase compared to docetaxel alone group) (Fig. 38). Area under the curve for docetaxel was increased by 230% in the combination group as against docetaxel alone group. Further, $t_{1/2}$ of docetaxel increased from 0.44 h to 1.14 h in piperine-docetaxel combination group.

Data from the xenograft model suggested a significant decrease in the growth of tumors in docetaxel-treated group (313% vs. 461%, p=0.039) after two weeks of treatment. An evident decrease in tumor growth was also witnessed in piperine only group (373% vs. 461%, p=0.201). Most significant tumor inhibition was observed (188% vs. 461%, p=0.003) in animals treated with the combination of piperine and docetaxel (Fig. 39). Furthermore, mean docetaxel plasma level increase in the combination group as a result of piperine treatment did not produce any observable toxicity in mice during the study. Also, no premature death was witnessed in treatment groups during the study.

Overall, these findings suggest that piperine could play a potential role in enhancing therapeutic efficacy of docetaxel in treating castration-resistant prostate cancer without increasing docetaxel-mediated toxicities (Makhov et al., 2012).

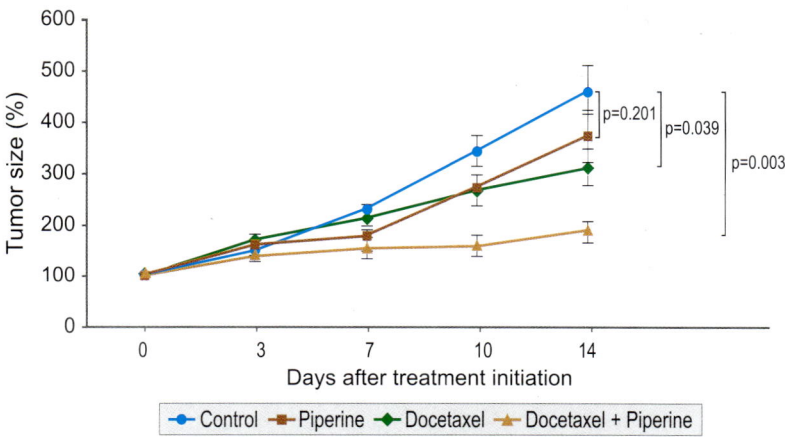

Fig. 39: Effect of piperine administration on antitumor efficacy of docetaxel.

Antitumor activities of piperine against androgen-dependent and androgen-independent prostate cancer, including underlying molecular mechanism were determined by Samykutty et al. In this study, it was shown that piperine inhibited proliferation and induced the cell death in human prostate carcinoma cells, including androgen-sensitive LNCaP and androgen-insensitive PC-3, 22Rv1 and DU-145 cells. Piperine (5–200 µM) produced a dose- and time-dependent (24–72 h) anti-proliferative effect against all cell lines. Piperine treatment (75 µM) in LNCaP cells also reduced prostate-specific antigen (PSA), the gold standard marker of prostate cancer, bringing its secretion to near normal levels (4.244 ng/ml) compared to untreated cells (41.24 ng/ml).

In addition, both Annexin-V FITC staining analysis and global caspase activation assay showed that anti-proliferative activity of piperine and cell viability are associated with apoptosis. Further experiments using LNCaP, PC-3 and DU-145 cells revealed that piperine treatment leads to caspase-3 activation and cleavage of Poly [ADP-ribose] polymerase 1 proteins. Piperine was also found to reduce the expression of NF-κB, STAT3 transcription factors and androgen receptor in LNCaP cells at 60 μM concentration. Anti-migration activity was also witnessed in LNCaP and PC-3 cells upon treating with piperine.

In vivo antitumor activity of piperine was determined using a xenograft model in nude mice using LNCaP (5×10^6) and DU-145 (1×10^6) cells, and were treated with piperine (100 mg/kg; i.p.) for one month. In a separate experiment, influence of piperine on the tumor growth was also studied by administering via oral gavage (10 mg/kg) after subcutaneous implantation of LNCaP cells. At the end of the experiment, tumors were excised from mice to measure mass and volume.

Piperine decreased the LNCaP and DU-145-derived tumor growth (tumor volume and tumor mass, both $p<0.05$) significantly by 72% and 41%, respectively in nude mice (Fig. 40A–D).

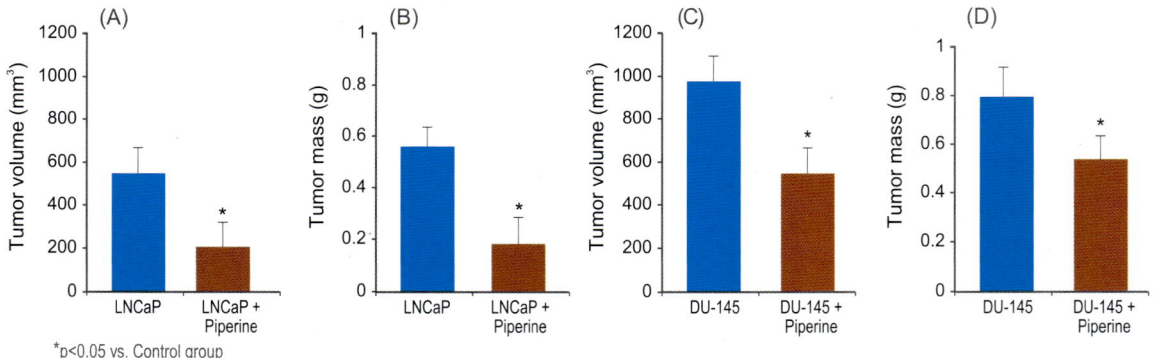

*$p<0.05$ vs. Control group

Fig. 40: Effect of piperine treatment on tumor growth in LNCaP- and DU-145-treated nude mice.

Importantly, oral administration of piperine was also found to exhibit significant tumor suppression activity in LNCaP-implanted mice (tumor volume and tumor mass, both $p<0.05$) (Fig. 41A and 41B).

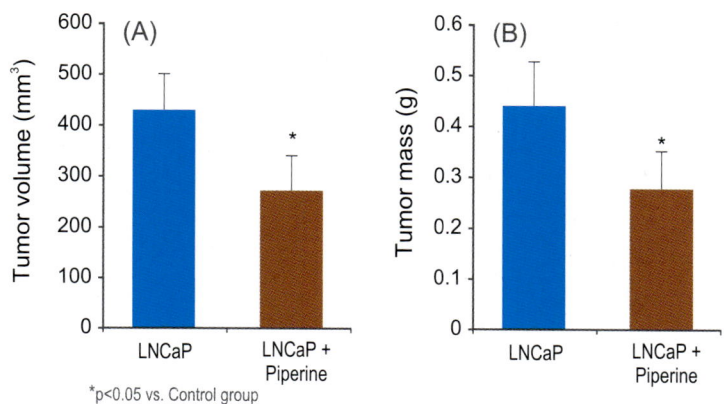

Fig. 41: Effect of oral administration of piperine on tumor growth in nude mice.

Based on these observations, it was concluded that piperine may be considered as a potential therapeutic agent in the treatment of prostate cancer (Samykutty *et al.*, 2013).

Chapter 4
PIPERINE AND ITS HEALTH BENEFITS

Management of Metabolic Syndrome

Metabolic syndrome is a cluster of complex clinical conditions, including hypertension, insulin resistance, high blood glucose levels, excess body fat and abnormal lipid levels, which increase the risk of cardiovascular diseases, stroke and diabetes. Worldwide, the prevalence of metabolic syndrome is on the rise mainly due to lifestyle changes and dietary habits with more than one third of the population being affected by the condition (Hollander and Mechanick, 2008; Roberts *et al*., 2013).

Change in lifestyle and diet are the first line of treatment for metabolic diseases. Although evidence-based interventions have been in practice since long to manage different aspects of the metabolic syndrome, natural approach to treat the condition could be very promising, as it is devoid of long-term adverse effects of the prescription medicines. In recent years, a number of innovative nutritional strategies have been proposed as safe and effective alternative treatments. Of these, dietary supplementation with piperine has been studied most extensively (Santini *et al*. 2017; Tabatabaei-Malazy *et al*., 2015).

A. Antidiabetic Activity

In vivo Studies

The effect of piperine on the pharmacokinetics and efficacy of glimepiride was studied in normal and streptozotocin-induced diabetic rat model by Veeresham *et al.* In diabetic mice, combination of glimepiride and piperine resulted in marked increase in pharmacokinetic parameters, such as C_{max}, AUC, $t_{1/2}$ and mean response time, and decreased clearance, V_d, compared to control group. Additionally, combination group showed improved antioxidant status in diabetic rats compared to individual treatment of glimepiride and piperine. Overall, it was suggested that piperine might be beneficial in diabetic patients as an adjuvant to glimepiride (Veeresham *et al.*, 2012). In glucose-challenged and alloxan-induced diabetic models, piperine administration along with nateglinide resulted in synergistic anti-hyperglycemic activity (Sama *et al.*, 2012).

In another study, antidiabetic effect of piperine was evaluated in alloxan-induced diabetic mice in acute and sub-acute models. Results suggested that sub-acute administration of piperine (20 mg/kg) produced statistically significant anti-hyperglycemic activity ($p<0.05$) (Atal *et al.*, 2012).

Recently, the same research group studied the bioenhancing effect of piperine with metformin on lowering blood glucose level in alloxan-induced diabetic mice. In this 4-week, sub-acute study, diabetic mice were divided into four groups and treated with standard metformin (250 mg/kg), piperine (10 mg/kg) combined with metformin at 250 mg/kg and 125 mg/kg, and untreated control. Blood glucose levels were estimated at day 0 (baseline), day 14 and day 28. Significant blood glucose lowering effects ($p<0.05$) were observed in groups treated with metformin and piperine combination compared to untreated as well as only metformin-treated groups on both day 14 and 28 (Atal *et al.*, 2016).

Antidiabetic potential of combination of curcumin with piperine and quercetin was evaluated in rat models of streptozotocin- and nicotinamide-induced diabetes. Results suggested that combination treatment significantly reduced the plasma glucose (Table 14), elevated the levels of LDL, cholesterol and TGs (Table 15), and improved the body weight when compared to diabetic control group after 28 days. Data from oral glucose tolerance test also revealed that combination group showing high glucose tolerance compared to diabetic control. Hence, it was concluded that combination of curcumin with piperine and quercetin could be effective in the management of type II diabetes (Kaur *et al.*, 2016).

Groups	Plasma Glucose Levels (mg/dL)				
	Baseline	Day 0	Day 7	Day 14	Day 28
Normal Control	84.5 ± 4.70	85.7 ± 3.57	85.4 ± 4.27	86.8 ± 4.30	87.5 ± 4.00
Diabetic Control	85.6 ± 3.88	254.4 ± 11.33	258.7 ± 11.8	261.8 ± 13.23	265.0 ± 13.31#
Diabetic + Glibenclamide (10 mg/kg/day)	93.6 ± 3.90	250.7 ± 10.5	193.5 ± 7.4*	166.6 ± 16.1**	120.6 ± 11.7**
Diabetic + CPQ extract (100 mg/kg/day)	86.8 ± 4.30	250.9 ± 13.3	210.9 ± 17.8*	171.5 ± 13.8**	123.1 ± 12.33**

Data are mean ± SEM; *p<0.05, **p<0.01 vs. Diabetic control group; #p<0.05 vs. Glibenclamide group
CPQ: Curcumin + Piperine + Quercetin combination

Table 14: Effect of combination of curcumin with piperine and quercetin on plasma glucose levels in diabetic rats.

Groups	Triglycerides (mg/dL)	Cholesterol (mg/dL)	LDL (mg/dL)
Normal Control	99.98 ± 7.19	94.63 ± 5.94	89.95 ± 9.62
Diabetic Control	207.61 ± 16.04#	142.8 ± 6.99#	151.10 ± 7.43#
Diabetic + Glibenclamide (10 mg/kg/day)	163.283 ± 11.40**	97.82 ± 5.29**	105.6 ± 8.50**
Diabetic + CPQ extract (100 mg/kg/day)	158.083 ± 10.07**	107.91 ± 8.4**	115.71 ± 10.03**

Data are mean ± SEM; *p<0.05, **p<0.01 vs. Diabetic control group; #p<0.05 vs. Glibenclamide group
LDL: Low-density lipoprotein; CPQ: Curcumin + Piperine + Quercetin combination

Table 15: Effect of combination of curcumin with piperine and quercetin on lipid profile in diabetic rats.

In another study by the same researchers, 100 mg/kg dose of combinatorial extract consisting of curcumin : piperine : quercetin in a ratio (94 : 1 : 5) was found to have potent antihyperglycemic and lipid lowering effects ($p<0.001$) in HFD rats who were administered with low-dose streptozotocin. Thus, it was concluded that this combinatorial extract could be an effective therapeutic agent in treating metabolic syndrome due to its potent antioxidant potential (Kaur and Meena, 2012).

Clinical Study

Recently, Panahi *et al.* evaluated antioxidant effects of bioavailability-improved Curcumin C3 Complex® in patients with type II diabetes, when co-supplemented with BioPerine®. In this 3-month, randomized, double-blind, placebo-controlled trial, 118 diabetic patients were randomized to receive Curcumin C3 Complex® (1000 mg/day) and BioPerine® (10 mg/day) or matching placebo.

Overnight fasting blood samples were collected at baseline and at the end of the study to evaluate change in oxidative indices (e.g. total antioxidant capacity, SOD activity and MDA levels). A significant increase in serum total antioxidant capacity and SOD activity (both $p<0.001$) was found, whereas serum MDA level was found to be significantly decreased ($p<0.001$) compared to placebo. Hence, it was concluded that co-supplementation of Curcumin C3 Complex® with BioPerine® produced a significant antioxidant impact in type II diabetic patients (Panahi *et al.*, 2017).

B. Blood Pressure Management

In vivo Studies

To explore the underlying mechanism(s) of cardiovascular effects of piperine, Taqvi *et al.* employed various animal models. In normotensive anesthetized rats, piperine produced a dose-dependent (1–10 mg/kg) reduction in the mean arterial pressure. In Langendorff's rabbit heart preparation, force and rate of ventricular contractions and coronary flow were partially inhibited by piperine. Piperine also inhibited high K^+ (80 mM) precontractions and partially inhibited phenylephrine—suggesting Ca^{2+} channel blockade, which was further confirmed when piperine treatment resulted in rightward shift in Ca^{2+} concentration-response curves. However, in Ca^{2+}-free medium, piperine (1–30 μM) produced vasoconstriction. In rat aorta preparation, piperine exhibited endothelium-independent vasodilator effect and was more potent than phenylephrine against high K^+ (80 mM) precontractions. In bovine coronary artery preparations, piperine completely inhibited high K^+ precontractions. Hence, it was concluded that blood pressure (BP) lowering effect of piperine is mediated possibly through Ca^{2+} channel blockade, whereas its vasoconstrictor effect helps restrict consistent decrease in BP (Taqvi *et al.*, 2008).

Another experiment carried out by Hlavačková *et al.* also corroborated the above findings on piperine's mechanism of action as antihypertensive agent. In this experiment, hypertension was induced in Wistar rats by administering N(G)-nitro-L-arginine methyl ester (L-NAME). Effect of 6-week piperine treatment was evaluated by measuring systolic BP every week. Additionally, specimens of thoracic aorta were processed to evaluate the effect of piperine treatment on media thickness, elastin, and smooth muscle cells actin and phosphotungstic acid hematoxylin, orecin and antibodies against iNOS. Study results showed that piperine decreased the rise in BP from the third week of treatment. Percentual and absolute content of phosphotungstic acid hematoxylin positive myofibrils and elastin content were also decreased by piperine treatment. Thus, it was concluded that piperine treatment led to partial prevention of rise in BP, probably by blocking voltage-dependent Ca^{2+} channels and supported by filamentous actin assembly (Hlavačková et al., 2010).

The same research group investigated the preventive effects of piperine and curcumin (individually as well as in combination) on BP increase and the pathological changes in blood vessel morphology in an animal model of hypertension.

Adult 12-week-old Wistar rats were treated with L-NAME (40 mg/kg/day) to induce hypertension for 6 weeks. Concomitantly, rats were either treated with piperine (20 mg/kg/day), curcumin (100 mg/kg/day) or the combination.

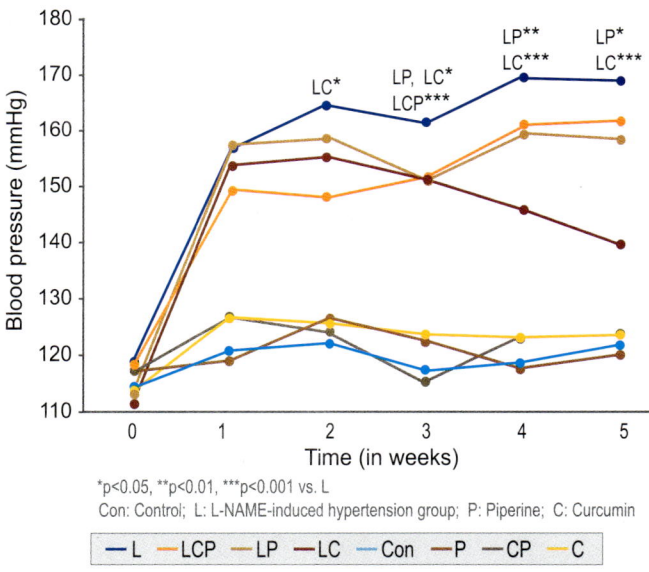

Fig. 42: Effect of piperine and curcumin treatment on L-NAME-induced blood pressure.

Systolic BP was measured weekly for 5 weeks and morphological changes in thoracic aorta were evaluated by histochemical analysis. Study results demonstrated that L-NAME induced an increase in BP after first week of administration, which exponentially increased each week. Piperine treatment resulted in significant reduction in BP compared to L-NAME-treated animals after three weeks. The combination of piperine and curcumin was also effective in reducing BP with statistical significance in week 3 (Fig. 42). Data from digital morphometry revealed that piperine was able to decrease the myofibrils content and slightly increase actin content in L-NAME-treated animals.

The combination showed significant reduction in the aortic wall thickness (i.e. cross section area, CSA) in hypertensive animals in comparison to L-NAME group (Fig. 43).

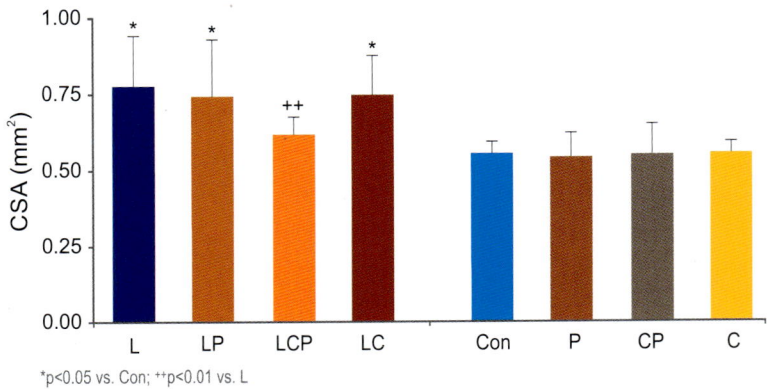

Fig. 43: Effect of piperine and curcumin treatment on changes in CSA of the media of aorta in hypertensive rats.

Overall, authors concluded that piperine was able to partially prevent increase in BP by L-NAME and associated negative changes (Hlavačková *et al.*, 2011).

C. Anti-obesity Activity

In vitro Studies

According to a recent study by Nogara *et al.*, increasing the metabolic rate of resting skeletal muscle could be an effective way of treating metabolic diseases like obesity and type II diabetes. In this experiment, researchers came up with a new mechanism of thermogenesis in skeletal muscles—i.e. variation in the ATPase activity of myosin, the motor protein.

Myosin has been known to exhibit two states: super-relaxed state (SRX) with the slower ATPase activity and the other one is disordered relaxed state (DRX) with the faster ATPase activity. Myosin heads spend most of their time in the SRX during low metabolic rate of resting skeletal muscle in both animals and humans. Hence, any agent that is able to shift the state of myosin heads from low metabolic rate to the high (i.e. from SRX to DRX) would in turn enhances thermogenesis. This would be beneficial in treating conditions like obesity and type II diabetes.

In the current study, a high-throughput screening of 2,128 compounds, including piperine, approved for human consumption by the Food and Drug Administration (FDA), was carried out using single-nucleotide turnover assay in skinned skeletal fibers. During the study, a fluorescent probe on a subunit of myosin, called regulatory light chain, showed an increase in emission intensity— suggesting transition of myosin heads from SRX to the DRX. The screen identified one compound, piperine, which was able to destabilize SRX.

Results demonstrated that piperine increased the ATPase activity of skinned relaxed fibers by 65 ± 15%. This phenomenon was only observed in fast twitch skeletal fibers (Fig. 44A) and not in slow skeletal fibers or cardiac tissues (Fig. 44B and 44C).

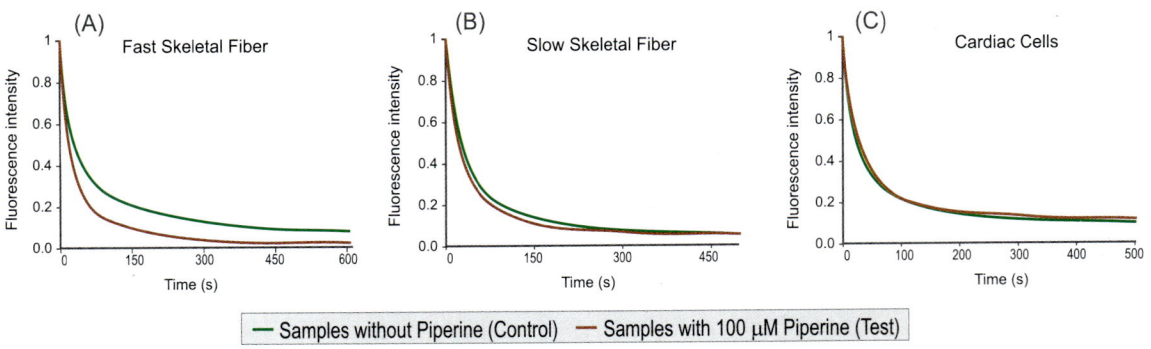

Fig. 44: Effect of piperine on metabolic rate of resting muscle fibers.

In conclusion, these results provided the proof of concept that piperine upregulates resting muscle metabolism, and thus could be an effective therapeutic option in treating obesity and type II diabetes (Nogara et al., 2016).

Anti-adipogenic activity of black pepper extract and piperine, and the underlying mechanism were evaluated in 3T3-L 1 preadipocytes. Adipocyte differentiation of 3T3-L 1 cells was significantly inhibited by both black pepper extract and piperine without affecting the cell viability. A marked reduction in mRNA expression of the master adipogenic transcription factors, peroxisome proliferator-activated receptor-gamma (PPAR-γ), sterol regulatory element-binding protein 1c, CCAAT-enhancer-binding protein-beta was also observed. Piperine significantly inhibited rosiglitazone-induced PPAR-γ transcription as well as disrupted rosiglitazone-dependent interaction between PPAR-γ and co-activator, CBP. Overall, it was further observed that piperine regulated the genes associated with lipid metabolism. It was concluded that piperine could be useful in treating obesity-related conditions (Park et al., 2012).

The role of spice-derived phytochemicals, including piperine in obesity-induced inflammatory response was studied using mesenteric adipose tissue isolated from high-fat diet (HFD) induced obese mice. Chemotaxis assay results revealed a concentration-dependent inhibition of degree of macrophage migration. It suggested that piperine suppressed obesity-induced inflammatory responses by suppressing adipose tissue macrophage accumulation or activation, and by inhibiting release of MCP-1 from adipocytes. Thus, spice-derived components like piperine can be potential candidates to address chronic inflammatory conditions in obesity (Woo et al., 2007).

In vivo Studies

Anti-obesity effects of piperine on HFD-induced obesity in rats were investigated by BrahmaNaidu *et al*. Different doses of piperine (20–40 mg/kg) were administered for 42 days and various parameters like changes in body weight, body composition, fat percentage, adiposity index, BP, plasma levels of glucose, insulin resistance, leptin, adiponectin, plasma and tissue lipid profiles, liver antioxidants along with activities of lipase, amylase and lipid metabolic marker enzymes, such as HMG-CoA reductase, carnitine palmitoyl transferase, fatty acid synthase, acetyl-CoA carboxylase, lecithin-cholesterol acyltransferase (LCAT) and lipoprotein lipase were assessed in experimental rats. A dose-dependent reversal of HFD-induced alterations (e.g. total fat, adiposity index) was observed with 40 mg/kg piperine showing significant activity ($p<0.05$) (Fig. 45A and 45B). Hence, it was concluded that piperine can be considered as an effective bioactive molecule to suppress body weight, improve insulin and leptin sensitivity, thus eventually regulating obesity (BrahmaNaidu *et al.*, 2014).

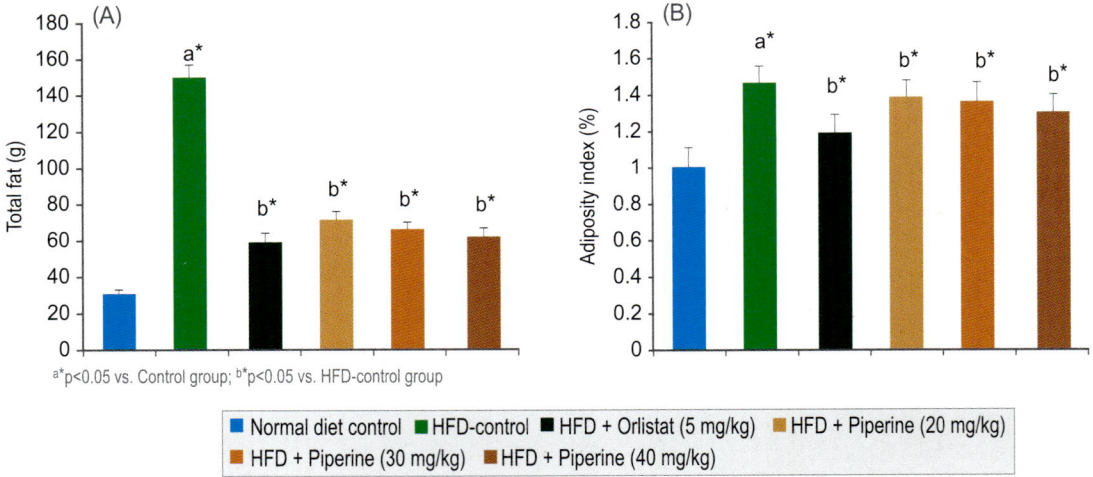

Fig. 45: Effect of piperine on (A) Total fat (B) Adiposity index in HFD-fed rats.

In another study, beneficial effect of piperine in obesity-induced dyslipidemia was evaluated. Male SD rats were fed either with HFD for 8 weeks followed by treatment with piperine (40 mg), sibutramine (5 mg), as standard treatment, or left untreated and continued on HFD until 11 weeks. Rats fed with normal diet served as control. Various parameters like body weight, biochemical parameters (serum TG and serum glucose) and insulin tolerance test were carried out at different time points. At the end of the study, fat mass was collected from each group (n=5) and weighed immediately.

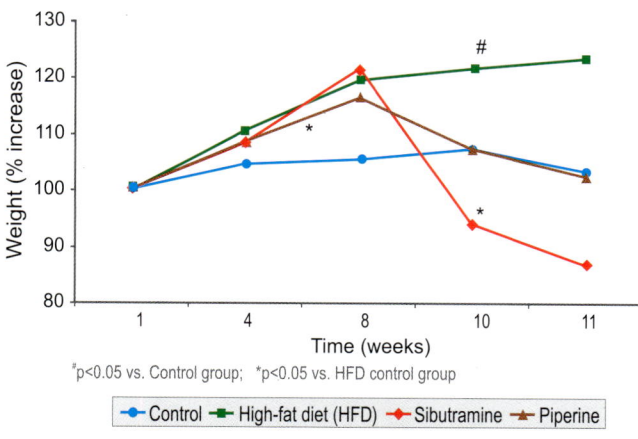

Fig. 46: Effect of piperine on body weight of high-fat diet animals.

Animals fed with HFD showed an increase in the body weight compared to control for the first 8 weeks. Piperine and sibutramine treatment resulted in significant decrease in the body weight ($p<0.05$) compared to untreated group (Fig. 46). Similarly, three weeks of piperine treatment showed significant decrease in serum TG, serum glucose levels and insulin sensitivity compared to HFD control group ($p<0.05$). The protective role of piperine was also observed during fat pad analysis. A significant reduction in the epididymal (visceral white adipose tissue, WAT) and interscapular (brown adipose tissue) fat mass was witnessed in piperine-treated group in comparison to HFD control group

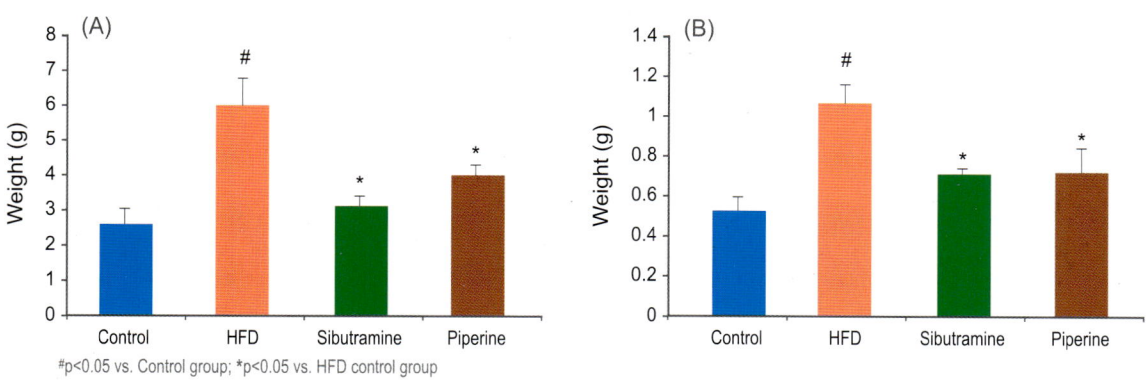

Fig. 47: Effect of piperine on (A) Epididymal fat mass (B) Interscapular fat mass in high-fat diet animals.

(p<0.05) (Fig. 47A and 47B). In conclusion, piperine exhibited significant anti-obesity, antidiabetic activity as well as improved insulin sensitivity in HFD-fed rats (Shah et al., 2010).

Energy metabolism enhancement following suppression of body fat accumulation by piperine was evaluated *in vivo* by Okumura *et al*. To confirm the action of piperine, the suppressive effect of black pepper on body fat accumulation was also investigated. In this study, C57Bl/6 male mice were fed with high-fat, high-sucrose diet for 4 weeks to induce adiposity. Results suggested that there was no difference in total food intake and total energy intake between control and piperine-treated group. However, a significant decrease in the body weight was observed in group treated with 0.05% piperine (Fig. 48). Additionally, values of serum components (e.g. glucose, TGs, total cholesterol and non-esterified fatty acids) were not significantly different between treated groups.

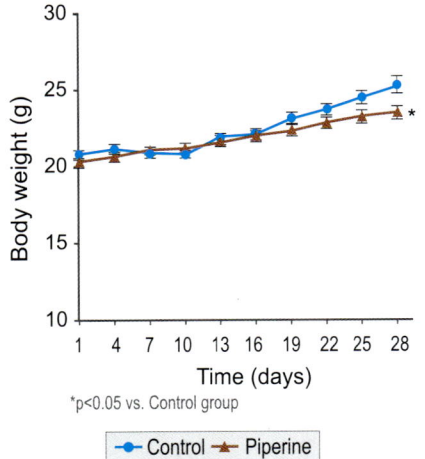

Fig. 48: Effect of piperine on body weight in obese mice.

Data from visceral fat weights analysis also suggested that piperine significantly suppressed the body fat accumulation. Piperine treatment was found to significantly reduce mesenteric, perinephric and epididymal WAT weights, with mesenteric WAT weight being decreased

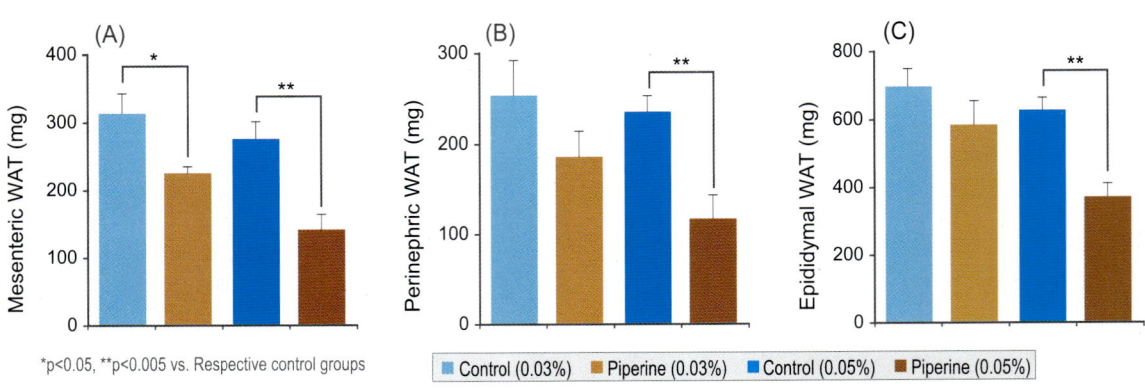

Fig. 49: Effect of piperine on visceral fat weights (A) Mesenteric (B) Perinephric (C) Epididymal in obese mice.

significantly in both the groups treated with piperine (0.03% and 0.05%), while 0.05% piperine decreased perinephric and epididymal WAT weights (Fig. 49A–C).

Similar results were seen when suppressive effect on body fat accumulation by black pepper extract was evaluated. At the end of week 4, concomitant supplementation of black pepper extract with HFD produced significant reduction in the body weight. Visceral adipose tissues weight was also significantly decreased by black pepper extract treatment, thus suggesting that black pepper extract suppresses adiposity (Okumura et al., 2010).

Clinical Study

In a randomized, double-blind, placebo-controlled, 8-week trial, efficacy of combination of bioactive food ingredients, including piperine on metabolic changes in overweight individuals was carried out. The study involved 103 eligible subjects who were randomly assigned to either supplemented group [n=41; 26 women, 15 men; age: 43.7 ± 8.5 years; body mass index (BMI) = 30.3 ± 3.5 kg/m^2] or placebo group (n=45; 29 women, 16 men; age: 40.7 ± 10.2 years; BMI = 30.0 ± 2.7 kg/m^2).

Evaluation of parameters that changed by intake of combination of bioactive food ingredients for eight weeks included: i) body composition, as the primary endpoint, ii) satiety control, iii) thermogenesis, iv) serum markers of lipolysis (free fatty acids and glycerol), v) adipokine release (leptin and adiponectin), vi) C-reactive protein (CRP) and insulin resistance, vii) angiogenesis marker release (vascular endothelial growth factor, VEGF) and viii) urinary norepinephrine. Additionally, Short-Form 36-Item Health Survey was conducted to assess health-related quality of life.

Twelve hours fasting blood samples were taken for the routine biochemical analysis measurements and other required parameters. To assess norepinephrine, 24 h urine test was also carried out. The same parameters were assessed after 8 weeks of treatment with either dietary supplement (2 capsules per day) or placebo.

Results indicated that there was no significant difference between supplemented group and the control group in terms of baseline characteristics. A significant difference between treatment groups was observed for the following parameters: insulin levels (p=0.003), insulin resistance [assessed by homeostasis model assessment, HOMA (p=0.002) and QUICKI, a quantitative insulin-sensitivity check index, (p=0.007)], leptin/adiponectin ratio (p=0.40), respiratory quotient (RQ) (p=0.008), LDL-cholesterol levels (p=0.031) and urinary norepinephrine levels (p<0.001) (Table 16). Compared to baseline values, a significant reduction in leptin, ghrelin and CRP, and an increase in thermogenesis (by 120 kcal/die) was observed in piperine-supplemented group, while significant decrease in adiponectin levels

Parameters	Supplemented group (mean change[a])	Placebo group (mean change[a])	p value
Insulin (pmol/L)	1.8	0.11	0.003
Insulin resistance			
i. HOMA	0.42	0.02	0.007
ii. QUICKI	− 0.01	0.00	0.002
Leptin/Adiponectin ratio	0.46	− 0.54	0.04
Respiratory Quotient (RQ)	0.04	− 0.04	0.08
LDL-cholesterol (mmol/L)	− 4.9	6.6	0.013
Urinary norepinephrine (nM/24 h)	− 24.6	5.0	<0.001

[a]Within-group changes are calculated as baseline − final value. Thus, a plus sign (+) corresponds to higher values at baseline (or a decrease during follow-up) and a minus sign (−) to lower values at baseline (or a increase during follow-up)

HOMA: Homeostatic model assessment; QUICKI: Quantitative insulin-sensitivity check index; LDL: Low-density lipoprotein

Table 16: Effect of combination of bioactive food ingredients on biochemical and urinary parameters.

were observed in placebo. Piperine-supplemented group also showed significant changes in BMI, fat mass, thermogenesis/free fat mass and VEGF but not in the placebo group. There were no significant changes observed for other parameters evaluated, viz. blood chemistry, anthropometric parameters, sense of satiety and quality of life survey.

Overall, it was concluded that combination of bioactive supplements comprising piperine might be helpful in the management of obesity-related inflammatory metabolic dysfunctions by reducing insulin resistance and inflammatory adipokines (Rondanelli *et al.*, 2013).

D. Antihyperlipidemic Activity

In vitro Studies

Duangjai *et al.* conducted a study to compare the effects of both black pepper extract and piperine on i) cholesterol uptake and efflux, ii) membrane/cytosolic distribution of cholesterol transport proteins and iii) physicochemical properties of cholesterol micelles in Caco-2 cells. Results suggested that both black pepper extract (containing same amount of piperine) and piperine decreased the cholesterol uptake into Caco-2 cells in a dose-dependent manner. Both preparations also reduced membrane levels of cholesterol transport proteins. Hence, these data suggested that piperine reduces cholesterol uptake by internalizing the cholesterol transport proteins (Duangjai *et al.*, 2013).

In a study conducted by Mueller *et al.*, out of 34 tested plant extracts, highest transactivation of PPARα, a nuclear receptor protein involved in various mechanisms that improve the lipid profile, was induced by piperine (EC_{50} = 84 µM). Thus, the study suggested that diet rich in herbs and spices like black pepper might be helpful in improving lipid profile, as they provide a number of PPARα agonists (Mueller *et al.*, 2011).

Influence of piperine on the expression of low-density lipoprotein receptor (LDLR) gene expression and consequent uptake of LDL-cholesterol into HepG2 cells was studied by Ochiai *et al.* In this study, food components, including piperine that stimulate LDLR gene promoter activity and their effect on proteolytic activation of SREBPs were studied by luciferase receptor gene assays.

Data showed that among tested compounds, piperine stimulated LDLR promoter activity and relative mRNA expression in HepG2 cells by more than 1.5-fold compared to control (Fig. 50A) in a concentration-dependent manner (Fig. 50B). Subsequently, piperine-mediated upregulation of LDLR mRNA led to enhanced LDL uptake in HepG2 cells after 5 h of piperine treatment.

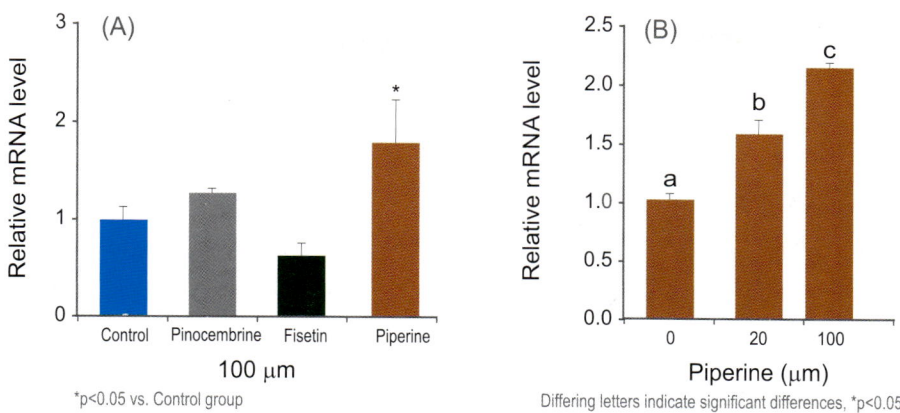

Fig. 50: Effect of piperine on LDLR mRNA expression in HepG2 cells.

Additionally, knockdown of SREBPs in HepG2 cells resulted in complete abolishment of piperine-mediated LDLR gene expression—thus, confirming that SREBPs are required to regulate LDRL gene expression.

Finally, the underlying mechanism of piperine in reducing serum cholesterol levels could be mediated by upregulation of LDLR gene expression and LDL uptake, which are further believed to be regulated by SREBPs (Ochiai et al., 2015).

In vivo Studies

Effective management of dyslipidemia in HFD-fed and antithyroid drug-induced hyperlipidemic rats was shown by piperine supplementation, as a dietary nutrient, by Vijayakumar and Nalini. In this study, rats were first divided into control and HFD group, which were then divided into four subgroups and treated with the following regimens for 10 weeks: i) control, ii) carbimazole (10 mg/kg), an antithyroid agent, iii) carbimazole + piperine (40 mg/kg) and iv) carbimazole + atorvastatin (2 mg/kg). Lipid profile, levels of hormones and apolipoprotein (Apo), a protein that plays a specific role in lipid metabolism, were evaluated.

Results demonstrated that animals treated with HFD and/or carbimazole showed significantly elevated plasma levels of total cholesterol, very low-density lipoprotein, LDL, TGs, free fatty acids and phospholipids, whereas high-density lipoprotein (HDL) levels were lower. In addition, treatment with carbimazole resulted in significant reduction in the levels of apo A1, T3, T4 and testosterone, while that of apo B, thyroid stimulating hormone and insulin were significantly elevated. However, piperine supplementation showed significant reduction in plasma lipids and lipoprotein levels, except HDL levels, which were found to be elevated. Additionally, plasma levels of apo A1, T3, T4 and testosterone were increased significantly, while apo B, thyroid stimulating hormone and insulin levels were brought to normal levels in treated animals. Hence, it was concluded that piperine exhibited potent thyrogenic activity as well as modulating effects on HFD-induced dyslipidemia in rodents (Vijayakumar and Nalini, 2006a).

The same group also demonstrated antioxidant efficacy of both black pepper extract and piperine in HFD-fed rats, wherein simultaneous supplementation with black pepper extract or piperine showed protection against tissue lipid peroxidation, thus reducing oxidative stress to the cells (Vijayakumar et al., 2004). Similar outcomes were witnessed in male Wistar rats, when piperine was supplemented concurrently along with HFD and antithyroid drug. Results indicated that by improving antioxidant status in hyperlipidemic rats piperine protected erythrocytes from oxidative stress (Vijayakumar and Nalini, 2006b).

Chapter 4
PIPERINE AND ITS HEALTH BENEFITS

In another study, Diwan et al. investigated the efficacy of piperine supplementation in high carbohydrate, high-fat diet-fed rats, a model of human metabolic syndrome. Study results suggested that supplementation with piperine (30 mg/kg/day) in high carbohydrate, high-fat-fed rats normalized the BP, improved the glucose tolerance and reactivity of aortic rings, decreased the oxidative stress and inflammation parameters, attenuated the inflammatory cell infiltration and fibrosis in cardiac and hepatic tissues, and improved the liver function (Diwan et al., 2013). Similarly, piperine showed beneficial effect by improving overall lipid profile in different hyperlipidemia models (Bao et al., 2013).

Cholesterol lowering potential of piperine and mechanism involved in preventing cholesterol gallstones formation were assessed in C57Bl/6 mice fed with LD containing high cholesterol levels. Results demonstrated that 10 weeks of concomitant supplementation with piperine (15, 30 and 60 mg/kg) resulted in decreased crystals in bile and improved serum lipid profile (i.e. lower total cholesterol, TGs and higher HDL:LDL ratio). Furthermore, piperine treatment reduced the liver lipid peroxidation as well as rendered protection from liver injury by improving SOD and inhibiting MDA levels. In addition, inhibitory effect of piperine on expression of ATP-binding cassette transporters G5/8 and liver X receptor (LXR) in liver as well as decreased cholesterol transportation from the hepatocytes to the gallbladder was thought to be the mechanism involved in the prevention of cholesterol gallstones formation (Song et al., 2015).

Protective effects of piperine against hepatic steatosis and insulin resistance, and the underlying mechanisms involved were explored by Jwa et al. A dose-dependent inhibition of ligand-induced LXRα activity by piperine was seen.

In HFD-fed mice supplemented with piperine (0.05%), a significant reduction in body and liver weight as well as plasma and hepatic lipid levels was observed. In addition, dietary piperine was found to markedly decrease mRNA expression of LXRα along with its different lipogenic target genes. Piperine was also found to significantly reduce the concentration of insulin and glucose, while increasing insulin sensitivity in HFD-fed mice and reduced endoplasmic reticulum stress. Overall, regulation of lipogenesis, which in turn influenced the hepatic lipid accumulation, was probably due to alterations in LXRα transcriptions (Jwa et al., 2012).

Recently, comparative beneficial effects of piperine and simvastatin in the treatment of hepatic steatosis were evaluated in hyperlipidemic rats. Hyperlipidemia was induced in male Wistar rats by feeding them with a cholesterol mixture every day for 8 weeks. Animals were divided into 4 groups, viz. control, high-fat, high-fat+piperine (40 mg/kg) and high-fat+simvastatin (2 mg/kg), and were treated concurrently 8 h after feeding with cholesterol mixture.

Parameters like liver cholesterol, TG, TBARS, SOD, serum aspartate aminotransferase and alanine aminotransferase were measured at the end of the experiment. Piperine treatment resulted in significant decrease in the accumulation of cholesterol, TG and lipid peroxidation in the liver, whereas activity of SOD was elevated. In comparison to high-fat group, activities of aspartate aminotransferase and alanine aminotransferase were significantly decreased in high-fat+piperine group.

This protective effect of piperine against fat accumulation in the liver could be due to the inhibition of pancreatic lipase activity and improved antioxidative status, as suggested by *in vitro* experiment (Tunsophon and Chootip, 2016).

Hypocholesterolemic effect of co-administration of curcumin with piperine was evaluated in HFD-fed rats by Tu *et al*. In this study, male SD rats were randomly divided into five groups and were fed with either normal diet or HFD containing 10% fat and 2% cholesterol for 8 weeks. Following 5 weeks, normal diet-fed (normal control, N) and HFD-fed rats (HFD control, H) were treated with corn oil, whilst other HFD-fed rats were treated with curcumin (100 mg/kg) (C group), piperine (5 mg/kg) (P group) or co-administered curcumin with piperine (CP group) for 4 weeks.

At the end of the study, lipid levels (total cholesterol, TG, HDL-cholesterol, LDL-cholesterol, ApoA 1, ApoB and total bile acid) were measured in serum, liver and fecal samples. Measurement of LCAT activity in serum and cholesterol 7α-hydroxylase (CYP7A1) activity in the liver was also done. Additionally, gene expression of ApoA 1, LCAT, CYP7A1 and LDLR was studied by qPCR analysis of hepatic samples.

Results suggested that co-administration of curcumin with piperine significantly lowered the levels of total cholesterol, TG and LDL-cholesterol in serum and liver, while the levels of HDL-cholesterol and ApoA 1 were increased (Table 17 and 18). Fecal levels of total cholesterol, TG and TBA were increased in combination group (Table 18).

Parameter	N	H	H+CP
TC (mmol/L)	4.02 ± 0.96	7.16 ± 1.59[b]	4.52 ± 1.36[c]
TG (mmol/L)	1.94 ± 1.05	4.28 ± 1.17[b]	1.96 ± 1.33[c]
HDL-C (mmol/L)	2.85 ± 0.58	1.70 ± 0.16[a]	2.88 ± 0.46[c]
LDL-C (mmol/L)	1.16 ± 0.66	5.34 ± 0.52[b]	1.64 ± 0.77[c]
ApoA 1 (g/L)	0.063 ± 0.006	0.018 ± 0.006[b]	0.064 ± 0.011[c]
ApoB (g/L)	0.075 ± 0.017	0.112 ± 0.010[a]	0.107 ± 0.012

[a]$p<0.05$, [b]$p<0.01$ vs. N group; [c]$p<0.01$ vs. H group
HDL-C: High-density lipoprotein cholesterol; LDL-C: Low-density lipoprotein cholesterol;
ApoA 1: Apolipoprotein A1; ApoB: Apolipoprotein B

Table 17: Effects of combination of piperine and curcumin on the serum lipid levels in HFD-fed rats.

Parameter	N	H	H+CP
TC (μmol/g liver)*	9.97 ± 3.12	34.76 ± 4.31[b]	12.52 ± 2.27[c]
TG (μmol/g liver)*	17.26 ± 3.78	40.35 ± 4.84[b]	22.56 ± 3.44[c]
TC (μmol/g of feces/day)[#]	5.69 ± 1.47	11.10 ± 2.29[b]	17.33 ± 3.16[c]
TG (μmol/g of feces/day)[#]	1.71 ± 0.36	3.84 ± 2.25[b]	7.05 ± 2.40[c]
TBA (μmol/g of feces/day)[#]	169.21 ± 30.8	218.10 ± 16.65[a]	266.44 ± 29.43[c]

*Hepatic lipids and [#]Fecal lipids. [a]$p<0.05$, [b]$p<0.01$ vs. N group; [c]$p<0.01$ vs. H group
TC: Total cholesterol; TG: Triglyceride; TBA: Total bile acid
N: Normal control; H: HFD control; C: Curcumin (100 mg/kg); P: Piperine (5 mg/kg)

Table 18: Effects of combination of piperine and curcumin on hepatic and fecal lipid levels in HFD-fed rats.

Combination treatment also resulted in marked increase in the serum LCAT and hepatic CYP7A1 activities compared to HFD control or curcumin alone. Furthermore, analysis of hepatic mRNA levels using qPCR showed that combination group produced a significant upregulation of gene expression of ApoA 1, CAT, CYP7A1 and LDLR compared to curcumin alone.

Overall, these results indicated that co-administration of curcumin with piperine could be promising in treating hyperlipidemia condition (Tu et al., 2014).

Neuropharmacological Effects

The brain is probably the most stressed organ in the human body due to current lifestyle and work pattern. It is a very complex, sensitive organ, which needs to be nourished in order to function properly. Over the time, the build-up of toxins in the body from pollutants, drugs and free radicals might interfere with the due cellular processes of the brain. Hence, disorders of the brain are considered, globally, as a major health challenge of the 21st century. Research during the past decade has provided stronger evidence suggesting that frequency and burden of these diseases is much more than previously thought (Wattanathorn *et al.*, 2008; Wittchen *et al.*, 2011).

In such a scenario, demand for natural ingredients that help support nervous system significantly is ceaseless. Piperine is one such natural active principle that has been known for its merits in maintaining optimal brain health and functioning. Several studies have corroborated beneficial role of piperine on the nervous system as a whole.

Chapter 4
PIPERINE AND ITS HEALTH BENEFITS

A. Cognitive Enhancing Effects

In vivo Studies

Neuroprotective role of piperine was observed in male Wistar rats when treated for 4 weeks. All doses of piperine (5–20 mg/kg) significantly decreased the escape latency (Fig. 51A) and increased the retention time (Fig. 51B) in Morris water maze test. Efficacy of piperine was comparable to that of donepezil, a standard drug. Thus, piperine has been shown to have cognitive enhancing effect at all dosage range (Wattanathorn *et al.*, 2008).

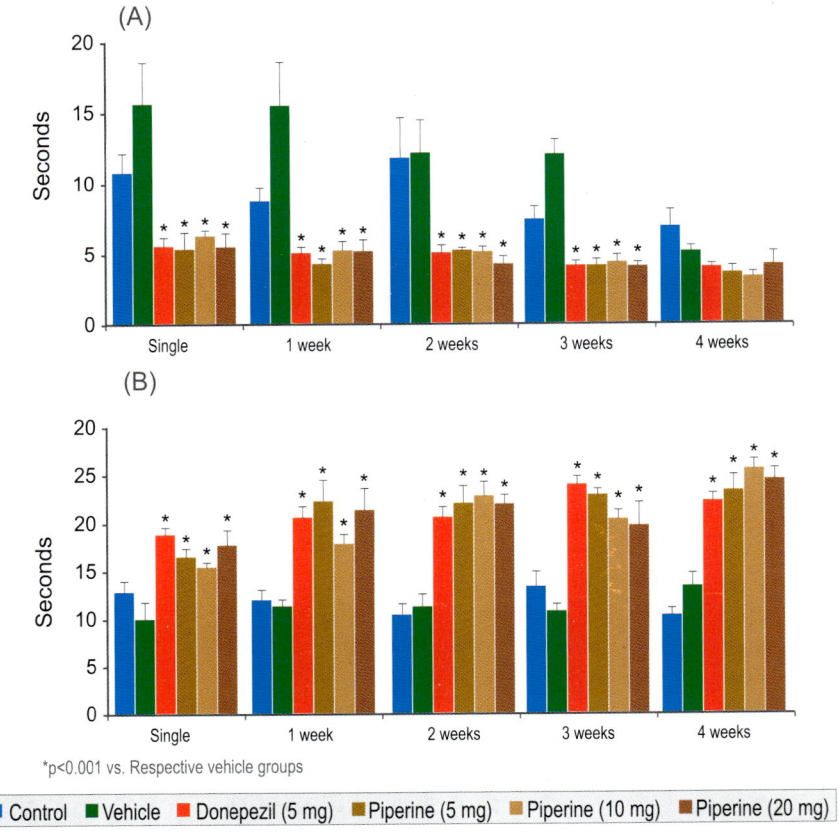

Fig. 51: Effect of piperine treatment on
(A) Escape latency (B) Retention time in Morris water maze test.

In another study, protective role of piperine against neurodegeneration and cognitive impairment in animal model of cognitive deficit-like condition of Alzheimer's disease was investigated by the researchers. Here, adult male Wistar rats were treated with piperine (5–20 mg/kg) 2 weeks before and a week after the intra-cerebroventricular administration of ethylcholine aziridinium ion (AF64A) bilaterally. At the end of the study, it was observed that piperine significantly inhibited memory impairment and neurodegeneration in hippocampus at all dosage range, possibly by inhibiting lipid peroxidation and acetylcholinesterase (AChE) enzyme activity. In addition, neuroprotective effect of piperine was also demonstrated (Chonpathompikunlert et al., 2010).

In a 28-day study, neuroprotective effects of quercetin in combination with piperine were evaluated in a mouse model of CUS-induced behavioral and biochemical alterations. Mice were subjected to a series of stressful events and were administered either quercetin (20–80 mg/kg), piperine (20 mg/kg) or the combination 30 min. prior to CUS procedure. Animals were assessed for various behavioral aspects using Morris water maze and elevated plus maze paradigms. Other biochemical parameters were also evaluated.

Co-administration of quercetin and piperine significantly restored behavioral, biochemical and molecular changes in stressed animals. In elevated plus maze task, transfer latency was significantly shortened, whereas considerable improvement in the retention of learning and memory was witnessed in the Morris water maze test (both $p<0.05$). Protective effect of the combination treatment was further supported by significantly decreased levels of MDA, nitrite concentration, restored GSH, SOD and catalase activity in combination group compared to individual treatment groups. Similarly, levels of AChE and corticosterone were significantly lowered upon combination treatment. Overall, it was concluded that co-administration of piperine with quercetin might be a helpful and effective adjuvant in the management of cognitive disorders (Rinwa and Kumar, 2013).

Effect of co-administration of piperine with curcumin against CUS-induced cognitive impairment and oxidative stress in mice was evaluated by the same group (Rinwa and Kumar, 2012). In this study, batteries of stressors were used to induce CUS in male LACA mice for

28 days. Mice were administered either vehicle, curcumin or curcumin-piperine combination daily 30 min. before CUS procedure.

Behavioral parameters evaluated for memory performance included Morris water maze (latency time to reach the platform), elevated plus maze test (latency time to reach the closed arm) and locomotor activity along with sucrose consumption test. Biochemical parameters, such as levels of MDA, GSH, catalase, AChE, serum corticosterone and nitrite concentration along with mitochondrial enzyme complex activities were measured to assess oxidative stress.

At the end of the study, it was found that chronic treatment with curcumin (200 and 400 mg/kg) significantly improved CUS-induced alterations in behavioral and biochemical parameters, restored mitochondrial enzyme complex activities and attenuated the elevated levels of AChE and serum corticosterone as well. However, significantly higher protective effects were observed when piperine (20 mg/kg; p.o.) was co-administered with curcumin (100 and 200 mg/kg; p.o.) in comparison to their effects alone. Hence, it was concluded that piperine potentiated the protective effects of curcumin against CUS-induced cognitive impairment and associated oxidative damage in mice (Rinwa and Kumar, 2012).

In another study, neuroprotective activity of simultaneous administration of piperine and curcumin alone and in combination against cognitive and motor impairment due to chronic exposure to D-galactose was studied in Wistar rats.

Young Wistar rats treated with D-galactose (150 mg/kg; s.c.) were simultaneously administered either piperine and curcumin alone or the combination for 56 days. Other groups included vehicle control, D-galactose alone and naturally aged control. At the end of the study, brain homogenates were evaluated for cognitive changes, motor impairment, protein carbonyls, protein thiols, advanced oxidation protein products, 4-hydroxynonenol and nitric oxide levels. Histopathological changes in the cerebellum were evaluated to determine motor performance.

Results showed that concurrent treatment with piperine led to cognitive enhancement, improved sensorimotor performance, decreased load of oxidative and nitrosative stress. Besides, combination treatment resulted in decreased alterations in the Purkinje cells. Hence, it was concluded that piperine could be an effective agent against age-related neurodegenerative disorders (Banji et al., 2013a).

The same group also hypothesized that piperine (12 mg/kg) and curcumin (40 mg/kg) could attenuate D-galactose-induced senescence and cognitive impairment in young adult male Wistar rats when treated for 49 days. This synergistic action was thought to be due to enhanced serotonergic signaling post-treatment (Banji et al., 2013b).

Chapter 4
PIPERINE AND ITS HEALTH BENEFITS

Clinical Study

A randomized, double-blind, placebo-controlled, cross-over study was carried out to ascertain whether co-supplementation of piperine with resveratrol affects the bioefficacy of resveratrol on cerebral blood flow parameters and cognitive performance in healthy adults. A total of 23 healthy adult volunteers (n=4, males; n=19, females) participated in all the three arms of this cross-over study. During three study visits, participants were given placebo, *trans*-resveratrol (250 mg) and combination of *trans*-resveratrol and piperine (20 mg) on separate days at least a week apart. Participants were asked to perform a selection of cognitive tasks before and after 40 min. of the treatment (i.e. after rest or absorption period), which was assessed in the frontal cortex using near-IR spectroscopy. Cerebral blood flow (CBF) was also assessed by measuring total hemoglobin levels. Bioavailability analysis was done in a separate cohort of volunteers (n=6).

The results indicated that compared to placebo and resveratrol alone, combination group showed significantly augmented CBF during most part of the task performance period (Fig. 52). Co-supplementation enhanced the bioefficacy of resveratrol with regard to CBF effects (Wightman *et al.*, 2014).

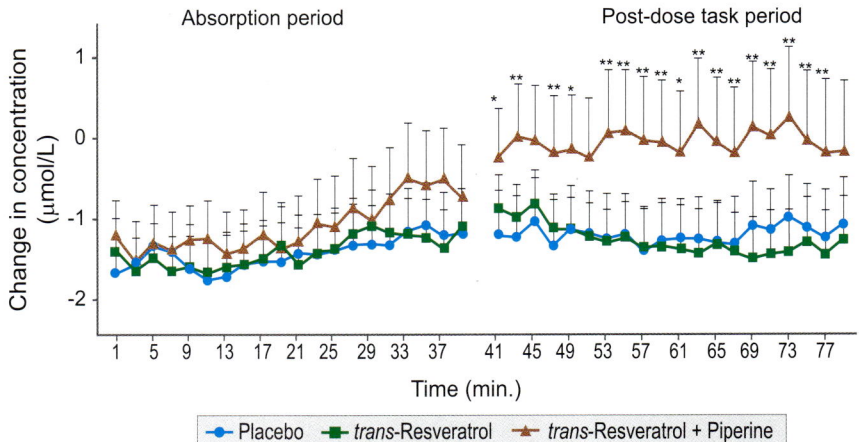

Fig. 52: Effects of co-supplementation of piperine with resveratrol on the concentration of hemoglobin in healthy volunteers.

B. Antidepressant and Anxiolytic Effects

In vitro Study

Neuroprotection is one of the most discussed mechanisms of antidepressants. Hence, neuroprotective role of piperine against corticosterone-induced neurotoxicity in cultured rat pheochromocytoma (PC12) cells was evaluated. Results proved that at 1 μM piperine had maximum inhibitory effect against cytotoxicity, while co-treatment also led to decreased intracellular ROS level, enhanced SOD activity and total GSH levels. Additionally, piperine treatment was able to reverse the decreased levels of brain-derived neurotrophic factor (BDNF) mRNA caused by corticosterone. Hence, it was concluded that neuroprotective benefits of piperine against corticosterone-induced neurotoxicity in PC12 cells could be due to inhibition of oxidative stress and the upregulation of BDNF mRNA (Mao *et al.*, 2012).

In vivo Studies

Effect of piperine on unpredictable chronic mild stress (CMS) rats as well as underlying mechanisms involving hypothalamic-pituitary-adrenal (HPA) axis were studied by Hu *et al*. Individually housed rats, exposed to CMS through unpredicted sequence of mild stressors were treated with different doses of piperine for 21 days. Change in body weight, sucrose preference test, serum levels of corticotrophin-releasing hormone, adrenocorticotropic hormone and corticosterone were evaluated at the end of the study. Piperine at 10 and 20 mg/kg dose increased the sucrose intake in CMS-induced rats, thus showing behavioral improvement. Serum levels of adrenocorticotropic hormone and corticotrophin-releasing hormone were significantly decreased by piperine in a dose-dependent (5, 10 and 20 mg/kg) manner. Overall, it was concluded that piperine can alleviate CMS-induced depression in rats by modulating the function of HPA axis (Hu *et al.*, 2009).

Antidepressant activity of piperine was assessed in rats using forced swim test (FST), wherein various parameters like immobility, climbing and swimming times were recorded during 5-minute test session at different time points. Results suggested a significant antidepressant activity (i.e. decreased immobility time and increased swimming time) with piperine treatment across all time points (Fig. 53A and 53B) and data were comparable to that of fluoxetine, a standard antidepressant (Wattanathorn *et al.*, 2008).

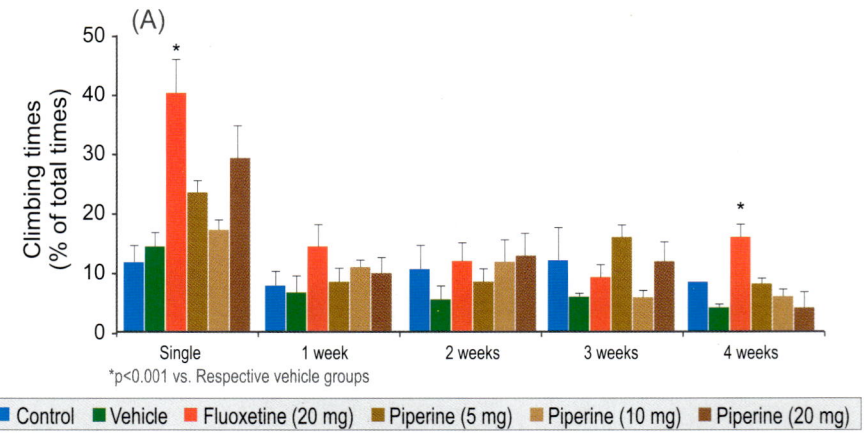

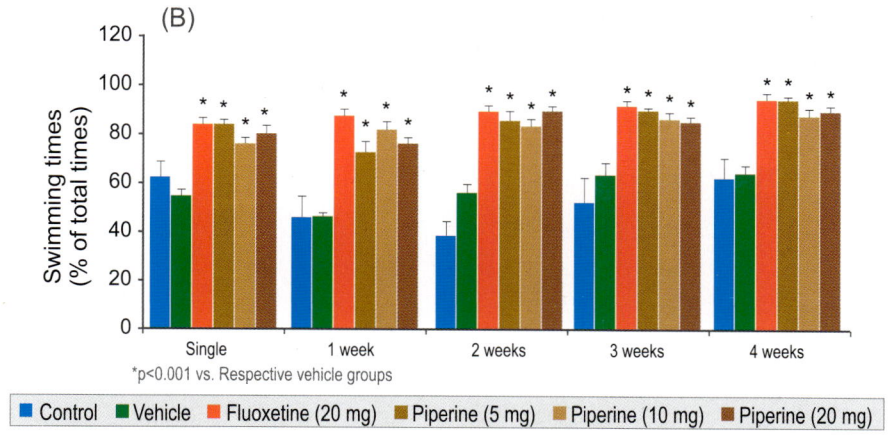

Fig. 53: Effect of piperine on
(A) Climbing time (B) Swimming time in forced swim test.

Several *in vivo* experiments carried out by Mao and team demonstrated that antidepressant activity of piperine is mediated by modulation of a number of signaling pathways.

Anti-immobility activity of piperine in different mouse models of depression proved its antidepressant-like effect. Involvement of serotonergic system was clearly demonstrated when piperine did not show its efficacy in mice pretreated with *para*-chlorophenylalanine (*p*CPA), a serotonin (5-HT) inhibitor. Number of head twitches following 5-hydroxytryptophan treatment, a metabolic precursor to 5-HT, was potentiated by piperine. Significant increase of 5-HT level in both the hippocampus and frontal cortex during neurochemical analysis further confirmed that antidepressant-like effect of piperine is mediated via serotonergic system by enhancing 5-HT content in the mouse brain (Mao *et al.*, 2011a). These findings were further confirmed when synergistic antidepressant effect was observed when mice were treated with sub-effective dose of piperine (1 mg/kg) along with 5-HT antagonist—suggesting that piperine's effects are mediated by the activation of 5-HT receptors (Mao *et al.*, 2011b).

Another set of experiments involving CMS-induced depressed rats suggested that piperine treatment significantly improved behavioral (increased sucrose intake, decreased immobility time in FST) and biochemical (increased levels of 5-HT and BDNF) changes —indicating that effects of piperine are mediated through pathways involving 5-HT and BDNF (Mao et al., 2014a). Similar results were observed in mouse models of depression (i.e. CMS- and corticosterone-induced depression), wherein chronic treatment of piperine (10 mg/kg) resulted in significant antidepressant activity in mice exposed to CMS and chronic corticosterone injections, and also demonstrated that BDNF signaling is vital for mediating piperine's effects (Mao et al., 2014b; 2014c).

Synergistic antidepressant-like effect was observed upon co-administration of sub-threshold dose of piperine (2.5 mg/kg) and low doses of *trans*-resveratrol (10 and 20 mg/kg) in *p*CPA-induced depression in mice as assayed by FST and tail suspension test, neurochemical (levels of monoamines in the frontal cortex, hippocampus and hypothalamus) and biochemical (monoamine oxidase activity) assays. Hence, it was concluded that antidepressant-like effects of this combination could possibly be due to positive modulation of monoaminergic system in the brain (Huang et al., 2013).

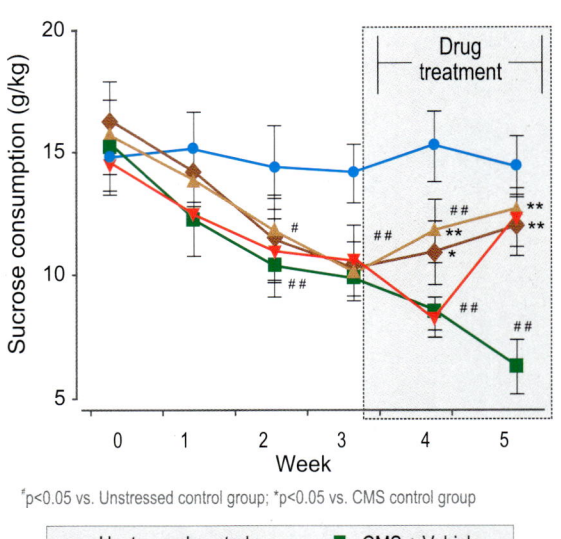

$^\#p<0.05$ vs. Unstressed control group; $^*p<0.05$ vs. CMS control group

Effect of piperine treatment in CMS-induced mice and possible mechanism involved was studied by Li *et al*. The study involved 14-day chronic, repeated administration of piperine (2.5–10 mg/kg) to mice subjected to CMS. Gradual recovery of sucrose intake was observed in CMS-induced animals treated with piperine; with higher sucrose consumption compared to fluoxetine group, a standard antidepressant (Fig. 54).

Fig. 54: Effect of piperine on sucrose consumption in CMS mice.

In a 5-minute open field test, locomotor activity of CMS mice was higher than non-stressed control group, especially during the first 2 minutes, while during the last 3 minutes it was lower. Furthermore, CMS mice showed more tendency towards center squares. Following 14 days of the treatment, the above mentioned behavioral changes in locomotor activity were reduced.

A separate group of animals was used to measure plasma corticosterone level. A higher corticosterone level was seen in CMS mice than in unstressed control group. The results indicated that antidepressant effects of piperine might be due to its ability to modulate HPA activity, and thereby resulting in neurogenesis. The elevated corticosterone level was significantly decreased after 2 weeks of repeated treatment with piperine (5 and 10 mg/kg) through 5 weeks (Table 19).

Group	Dose (mg/kg)	Corticosterone level (ng/ml)			
		Week 0	Week 1	Week 2	Week 5
Non-stressed	-	49.6 ± 6.3	47.8 ± 5.4	53.2 ± 4.9	48.4 ± 8.8
Chronic mild stressed (CMS)	-	47.8 ± 8.5##	165.3 ± 14.3##	153.1 ± 11.8##	75.6 ± 9.4#
Fluoxetine + stress	10	51.2 ± 7.6##	159.5 ± 13.4##	151.2 ± 13.9##	59.7 ± 6.4#**
	2.5	52.5 ± 6.6##	166.2 ± 15.2##	154.3 ± 13.1##	73.7 ± 8.2#
Piperine + stress	5	48.3 ± 7.9##	171.4 ± 16.6#	149.8 ± 17.4##	68.5 ± 8.4#*
	10	46.8 ± 5.7##	165.3 ± 12.9##	151.3 ± 13.1##	61.2 ± 6.9 **

#$p<0.05$, ##$p<0.01$ vs. Unstressed control group; *$p<0.05$, **$p<0.01$ vs. CMS group

Table 19: Effects of piperine on the plasma corticosterone level in CMS stressed mice.

Furthermore, piperine treatment decreased the proliferation of hippocampal progenitor cells, while the level of BDNF in the hippocampus of CMS group was upregulated. In addition, piperine (6.25–25 μM) dose-dependently protected primary cultured hippocampal neurons against the lesion induced by corticosterone (10 μM) as well as reversed the corticosterone-induced reduction of BDNF mRNA expression in cultured hippocampal neurons *in vitro* (Li et al., 2007).

In summary, the underlying mechanism of piperine's antidepressant-like effect could be due to its cytoprotective and neuroproliferating actions, which may be closely related to upregulation of BDNF level.

An attempt was made by Rinwa *et al.* to elucidate the neuroprotective mechanism of curcumin and its interaction with piperine against olfactory bulbectomy-induced depression in rats. Rats underwent bilateral olfactory bulb ablation and treatment was initiated after 14 days of surgical rehabilitation period.

Animals were treated with different doses of curcumin (100–400 mg/kg; p.o.), piperine (20 mg/kg; p.o.) or the combination once daily for another 2 weeks. Behavioral assessment involved FST, open field behavior and sucrose consumption test. This was followed by estimation of various biochemical, mitochondrial, molecular and histopathological parameters in the rat brain.

Results showed that removal of olfactory bulbs led to depression-like symptoms, which were evident from increased immobility time in FST, hyperactivity in open field arena and anhedonic-like response in sucrose consumption test, while significant alteration in mitochondrial enzyme complexes was seen along with increased serum corticosterone levels and oxidative damage. Additionally, other parameters like levels of inflammatory cytokines (e.g. TNF-α) and apoptotic factor (e.g. caspase-3) were elevated, whereas levels of BDNF were decreased. Histological abnormalities were also observed in olfactory bulbectomized rats.

However, treatment with curcumin significantly and dose-dependently restored all these behavioral, biochemical, mitochondrial, molecular and histopathological alterations in olfactory bulbectomized rats. Additionally, neuroprotective effects of curcumin (100 and 200 mg/kg) were further potentiated when co-administered with piperine (20 mg/kg) in comparison to individual treatment groups. For example, sucrose consumption in olfactory bulbectomized rats was significantly potentiated upon co-administration (Fig. 55A). Similar, effects were observed in case of BDNF levels. Combination of piperine (20 mg/kg) with curcumin (100 and 200 mg/kg) significantly elevated the levels of BDNF in olfactory bulbectomized rats (Fig. 55B).

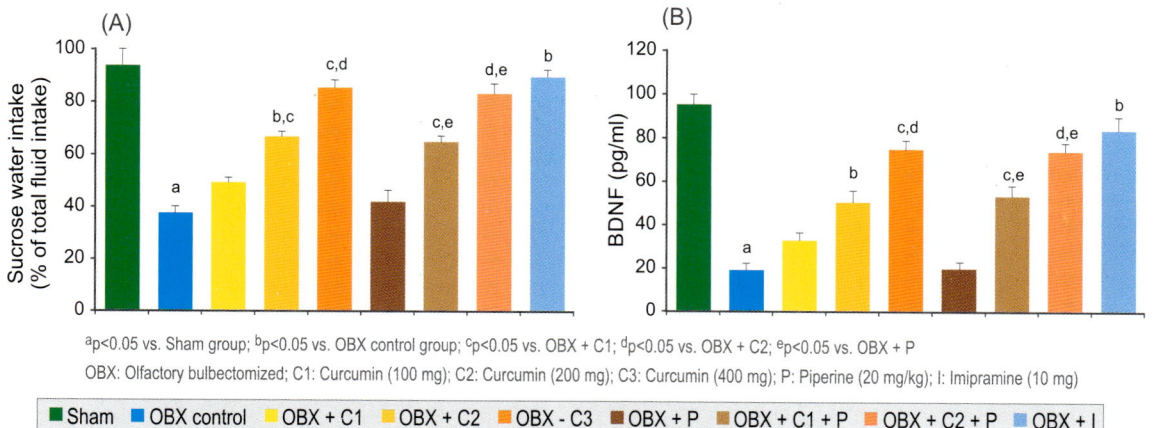

Fig. 55: Effect of co-administration of curcumin and piperine on (A) Sucrose consumption (B) BDNF levels in olfactory bulbectomized rats.

In conclusion, the current study highlighted that co-administration of curcumin and piperine may act as a useful natural adjuvant in the antidepressant therapy (Rinwa et al., 2013).

Possible anxiolytic activity and underlying role of γ-aminobutyric acid (GABA)ergic and nitriergic systems modulation of piperine were examined by Gilhotra and Dhingra in unstressed and stressed mice. Piperine treatment resulted in significant anti-anxiety activity in both unstressed and stressed (exposed to immobilization stress for 6 h) mice, which was comparable to diazepam, a standard anxiolytic agent. However, GABA levels were found to be elevated and no change in plasma nitrite levels in unstressed mice was observed. In stressed mice, piperine treatment did not cause any significant change in GABA levels, but marked decline in nitrite levels was observed.

Additionally, in unstressed mice pretreatment with 7-nitroindazole (20 mg/kg; i.p.), a neuronal NOS inhibitor, significantly potentiated the anxiolytic-like activity of piperine as compared to piperine and 7-nitroindazole alone groups. On the other hand, pretreatment with aminoguanidine (50 mg/kg; i.p.), an iNOS inhibitor, significantly enhanced the anxiolytic-like activity of piperine as compared to individual treatment of piperine and aminoguanidine in stressed mice. In conclusion, piperine exhibited anti-anxiety effects in unstressed mice possibly through GABAergic system and by inhibiting NOS, whereas the activity was through inhibition of iNOS in stressed mice (Gilhotra and Dhingra, 2014).

C. Anticonvulsant Activity

In vivo Studies

Piperine was shown to exhibit its anticonvulsant activity by blocking the convulsions induced by threshold doses of kainate (D'Hooge *et al.*, 1996), effectively by inhibiting synchronization of neural networks, modulating glutamate-mediated synaptic events and Ca^{2+} loading in cultured hippocampal neurons (Fu *et al.*, 2010), by activating TRPV1 receptor (Chen *et al.*, 2013) and by elevating the levels of 5-HT and catecholamine in different regions of E1 mice brain (Mori *et al.*, 1985).

In another study, $GABA_A$ receptor modulating effect of piperine was studied both *in vitro* and *in vivo*. Piperine demonstrated same level of potency on all $GABA_A$ receptor subtypes in oocytes of *Xenopus laevis*, while significantly increasing pentylentetrazole (PTZ) induced seizure threshold in mice at 3 and 10 mg/kg after 30 min. of the treatment (Khom *et al.*, 2013). Mishra *et al.* elucidated that piperine could modulate several neurotransmitter systems like 5-HT, norepinephrine and GABA via various *in silico*, *in vitro* and *in vivo* techniques. Overall data suggested that piperine's Na^+ channel antagonistic activity could be contributing to its complex anticonvulsant mechanisms (Mishra *et al.*, 2015).

In an animal model of pilocarpine-induced convulsions, effect of piperine alone and associated to other drugs like atropine, memantine, nimodipine, diazepam and flumazenil was evaluated. Additionally, its action on brain monoamine, amino acids and cytokines (e.g. TNF-α) were also studied. Male Swiss mice were acutely administered with piperine (2.5, 5, 10 and 20 mg/kg) followed by pilocarpine injection (350 mg/kg) after 30 min., whereas other drugs were administered 15 min. prior to piperine.

Behavioral testing involved assessment of piperine's effect on the development of convulsions followed by mortality rate and its effect after its association to aforementioned drugs. Results showed that latency to 1st convulsion was significantly increased by piperine in a dose-dependent manner compared to pilocarpine-treated group (Fig. 56A). Percentage of survivals 24 h after 1st convulsion and latency to death was increased from 58 to 138% (or decreased mortality rate) by piperine in a dose-dependent manner (Fig. 56B). Similar results were obtained in piperine group (1 and 2.5 mg/kg) pretreated with diazepam (0.2 and 0.5 mg/kg), while these effects were blocked by flumazenil (2 mg/kg), a benzodiazepine antagonist—suggesting involvement of GABAergic system.

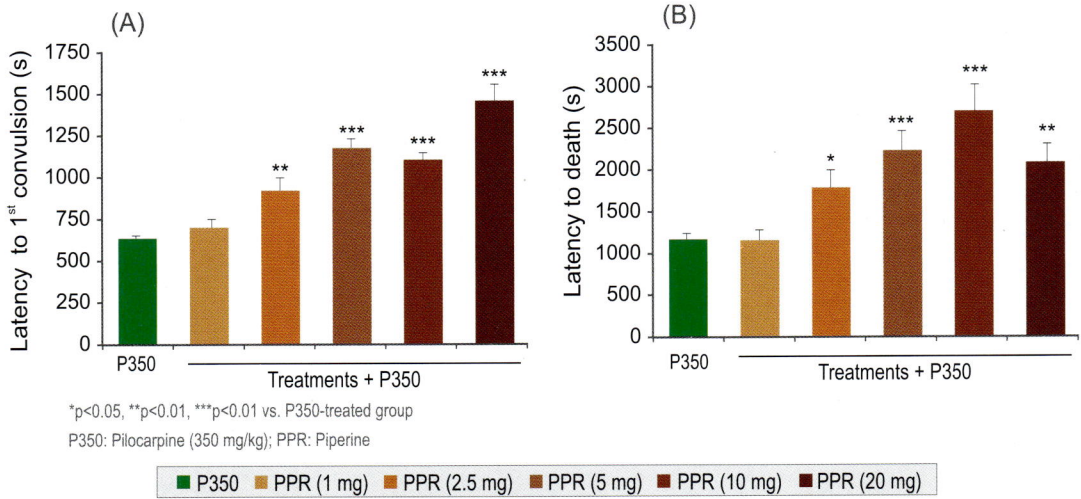

Fig. 56: Dose-dependent effect of piperine on (A) Latency to first convulsion (B) Latency to death.

Furthermore, piperine did not affect striatal levels of dopamine and its metabolites 3, 4-dihydroxyphenylacetic acid and homovanilic acid, while it increased the levels of GABA, glycine and taurine, and also reversed the increased levels of nitrite in pilocarpine group in sera and brain. Similarly, an increased number of TNF-α immunostained cells across hippocampi was observed in untreated pilocarpine group, which was found to be reversed in pilocarpine group pretreated with piperine.

In conclusion, piperine exhibits anticonvulsant action through multiple mechanisms, including its anti-inflammatory and antioxidant actions, in addition to its modulating effect on GABAergic system (da Cruz et al., 2013).

Recently, potential neuroprotective effect and efficacy of piperine in temporal lobe epilepsy or pharmaco-resistant epilepsy in pilocarpine model was studied by Pany *et al*. In this study, epileptic rats (induced by pilocarpine, 350 mg/kg) were treated for 30 days either with phenytoin (25 mg/kg), phenytoin+piperine (25 mg/kg each) or phenytoin (25 mg/kg)+ celecoxib (20 mg/kg). Naive animals treated with phenytoin served as control group. At the end of the study, animals were euthanized and blood and brain tissues were collected to estimate levels of phenytoin, measurement of lipid peroxidation, catalase activity, levels of GSH and neuronal cell count (% of viable neurons) in CA1 and CA3 regions of hippocampi.

Results indicated that co-administration of piperine as well as celecoxib with phenytoin significantly increased brain-plasma ratio of phenytoin, GSH level as well as % of viable neurons ($p<0.05$ all), while lipid peroxidation and catalase activity were remarkably decreased (both $p<0.05$). In summary, researchers concluded that piperine's potential neuroprotective effect and anticonvulsant activity may be attributed to its P-gp inhibition, COX-2 inhibition, Ca^{2+} channel blockade and inhibition of CYP3A4 enzyme activities (Pany *et al*., 2016).

In another study, protective role of piperine against epileptogenesis, cognitive impairment and oxidative stress was evaluated in PTZ-induced seizures in albino mice. Piperine at 2 and 4 mg/kg dose was found to significantly decrease PTZ-induced seizures and learning deficit (i.e. increased latency time and frequency of jerks) alone as well as when piperine (2 mg/kg) was co-administered with sodium valproate (300 mg/kg), a standard. Similar results were observed while assessing cognitive function through spontaneous alternation behavior test. Assessment of oxidative stress parameters also revealed that piperine alone (2 and 4 mg/kg) as well as in combination with sodium valproate significantly decreased whole brain MDA levels, whereas GSH levels were significantly increased.

Thus, it was concluded that piperine could be an effective adjuvant in preventing antiepileptic drugs-induced cognitive impairment (Rabbani and Ali, 2015).

Isobolographic and biochemical analysis of combination therapy of piperine and phenytoin in maximal electroshock-induced seizures model in mice also revealed the protective role of piperine against side effects associated with antiepileptic drugs therapy as well as synergistic potential of the combination against oxidative stress and improved brain 5-HT levels (Saraogi et al., 2013).

Effects of piperine on experimental models of convulsion, such as PTZ- and picrotoxin-induced seizures models were studied by Bukhari et al. In PTZ-induced model, mice were randomly treated with control, standard anticonvulsants (valproic acid, carbamazepine and diazepam) or different doses of piperine (30, 50 and 70 mg/kg) 30 min. before the induction of seizures by PTZ. In picrotoxin-induced seizures model, mice were pretreated with different doses of piperine or diazepam (1 mg/kg) 15 min. before the picrotoxin injection.

Results demonstrated that piperine produced a dose-dependent anticonvulsant activity compared to control group in PTZ model (Fig. 57A). Similar results were obtained from picrotoxin model, wherein piperine significantly increased the latency of convulsions in a dose-dependent manner when compared to control mice (Fig. 57B). Overall, it was suggested that anticonvulsant activity of piperine is possibly mediated via GABAergic pathway (Bukhari et al., 2013).

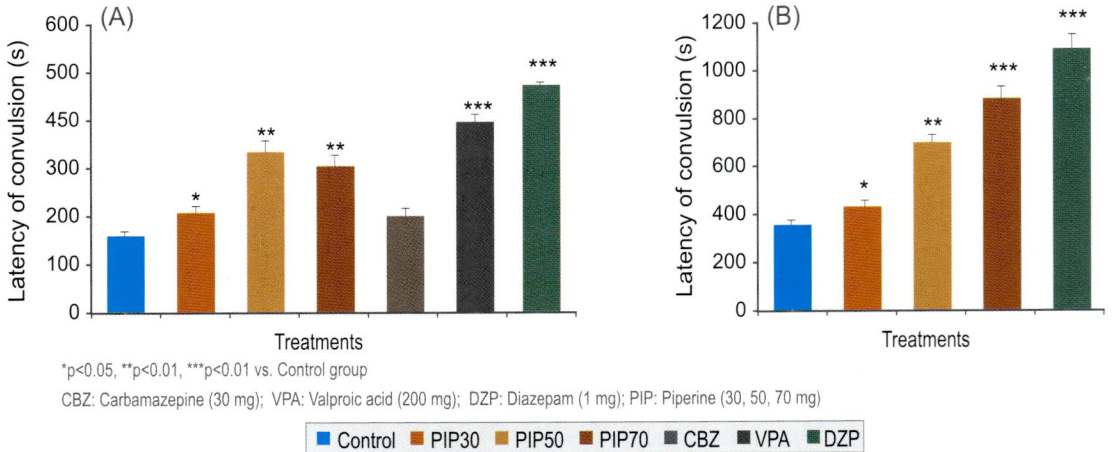

Fig. 57: Anticonvulsant activity of piperine in (A) Pentylenetetrazole Model (B) Picrotoxin Model for Seizures.

D. Antiparkinsonian Effects

In vivo Studies

Protective effect of piperine against 1-methyl-4-phenyl-1,2,3,6-tetrahydropyridine (MPTP) induced Parkinson's disease was evaluated in a mouse model. In this study, male C57bl/6 mice were administered with MPTP (30 mg/kg) for 7 days to induce Parkinson-like symptoms. Simultaneously, mice were treated with piperine (10 mg/kg) for 15 days (including 8 days of pretreatment).

Animals were evaluated for various behavioral and cognitive parameters using rotarod test (to assess motor co-ordination) and Morris water maze test (to assess cognitive impairments). After subjecting to these tests, mice brain samples were processed for immunohistochemical staining, estimation of MDA and SOD activity. In addition, microglial activation, expression of IL-1β and ratio of Bax: Bcl-2 were also assessed.

Results demonstrated that MPTP-induced decrease in the latency to fall off the rotarod was significantly attenuated by piperine (Fig. 58A). In Moris water maze test, piperine was able to protect against MPTP-induced cognitive impairment (e.g. spatial memory and learning ability). Data from immunohistochemistry suggested that piperine was able to protect dopaminergic neuronal death in substantia nigra pars compacta, a mid brain region predominant in dopamine neurons.

Additionally, piperine pretreatment resulted in significant reduction in the expression of IL-1β in the substantia nigra pars compacta of MPTP-treated brains, and alleviation of Iba-1, a marker of activated microglia—thus, advocating anti-inflammatory potential of piperine. Protective role of piperine against MPTP-induced oxidative stress was also witnessed when it significantly prevented the levels of MDA, whilst SOD activity was markedly improved.

Anti-apoptotic potential of piperine pretreatment was confirmed when it significantly alleviated decrease in the expression of Bcl-2 (anti-apoptotic protein) as well as attenuated increase in Bax (pro-apoptotic protein) expression in MPTP-treated mid brain samples (Fig. 58B).

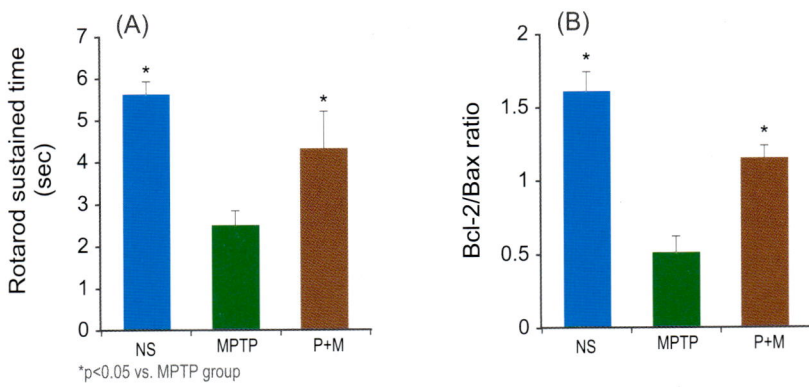

Fig. 58: Effect of piperine treatment on
(A) Motor co-ordination (B) Apoptotic signaling proteins.

Overall, results showed that piperine could be an effective treatment option for Parkinson's disease, owing to its protective role against MPTP-induced neurotoxicity, particularly on dopaminergic neurons (Yang et al., 2015).

Better neuroprotective effect of combination of piperine (2.5 mg/kg) with curcumin (25 mg/kg) against 6-hydroxy dopamine-induced Parkinson's rat model was observed by Singh and Kumar. Various parameters, viz. behavior, biochemical, neuro-inflammatory and neurochemical revealed promising results (Singh and Kumar, 2017). Furthermore, the same group has also demonstrated beneficial effects of chronic treatment with curcumin (25 mg/kg) and piperine (2.5 mg/kg) combination against 3-NP- (Singh et al., 2015) and QA-induced (a fungal toxin and excitotoxin, respectively) neurotoxicity in rats (Singh and Kumar, 2016). Twenty-one days of chronic treatment of the combination resulted in significant protection against motor deficit, biochemical and neurochemical abnormalities.

In another study, a formulation containing curcumin and piperine co-loaded glyceryl monooleate nanoparticles was found to exhibit augmented neuroprotection both *in vitro* and *in vivo* (Kundu et al., 2016).

Influence on Digestive System

According to a general perception, aromatic and pungent spices augment salivary and gastric secretions by imparting flavor and pleasing taste to the food that we eat (Srinivasan, 2009). In Ayurveda and other traditional systems of medicine, several preparations containing different spices have been recognized for their digestive-stimulant action and even used to manage digestive disorders.

However, these digestive effects of spices were largely empirical until recently, as several reports have now scientifically validated their beneficial role. Several studies have also demonstrated that spices induce enhanced secretion of bile acids and various digestive enzymes, which play a vital role in fat digestion and absorption. A few more studies have emphasized on the significance of spices in aiding accelerated digestion and reduction food transit time in the gastrointestinal tract, apart from their stimulant effect on either bile secretion or activity of digestive enzymes (Platel and Srinivasan, 2004).

Black pepper is one of the most widely used spices valued for its distinct role in supporting digestive process, primarily attributed to piperine. In the recent past, studies have shown that bioavailability enhancing ability of piperine is also partly attributed to its positive influence on absorption (Srinivasan, 2007).

A. Digestive Stimulant Activity

In vivo Studies

The influence of dietary intake of piperine on digestive enzymes of intestinal mucosa as well as that of pancreas was evaluated in experimental rats by feeding them with diet containing 20 mg% piperine (i.e. spice principle incorporated into the diet substituting an equal amount of corn starch) for 8 weeks. Results showed that piperine enhanced the activity of intestinal lipase, sucrase and maltase as well as stimulated the activity of pancreatic amylase, trypsin and chemotrypsin significantly (Platel and Srinivasan, 1996; 2000).

Another study by Bhat and Chandrasekhara demonstrated that black pepper when administered via oral gavage (250 mg) or diet-fed (0.2 and 0.4%) for 4 weeks caused an increase in bile solids secretion and increased bile flow, respectively (Bhat and Chandrasekhara, 1987a).

Clinical Study

In human subjects, Glatzel while studying the influence of spices on the secretion and composition of saliva, found that black pepper enhanced the secretion of saliva and salivary amylase activity (Glatzel., 1967).

B. Effect on Gastrointestinal Motility and Food Transit Time

In vivo Studies

Piperine was found to induce a dose- and time-dependent inhibition of GE of solids/liquids in rats, and the GT in mice. It was observed that piperine at 1 mg/kg showed significant inhibition of GE of solids in rats, whereas GT was inhibited at 1.3 mg/kg dose in mice. However, there was no effect on GE of liquids at the same dose. Overall, it was concluded that piperine's effect on GE is independent of gastric acid and pepsin secretion (Bajad et al., 2001). In another experiment, 6 weeks of dietary piperine intake produced a significantly shortened gastrointestinal food transit time (Platel and Srinivasan, 2001).

Effect of vanilloid ligands like piperine and anandamide on mice GT was evaluated by Izzo et al. Administration of piperine or anandamide (0.5–20 mg/kg) resulted in a dose-dependent shortening of GT. However, pretreatment of mice with capsaicin (75 mg/kg in total, 13 and 14 days before) significantly attenuated the inhibitory effect of piperine (10 mg/kg) on GT, but not that of anandamide (10 mg/kg) (Fig. 59). Hence, it was concluded that effects of piperine involves capsaicin-sensitive neurons, but not vanilloid receptors (Izzo et al., 2001).

These results (Izzo et al., 2001) were further corroborated when piperine reduced castor oil-induced intestinal fluid accumulation in a dose-dependent manner (2.5–20 mg/kg) in the mouse small intestine. This inhibitory action was strongly attenuated by capsaicin (75 mg/kg in total) (Capasso et al., 2002).

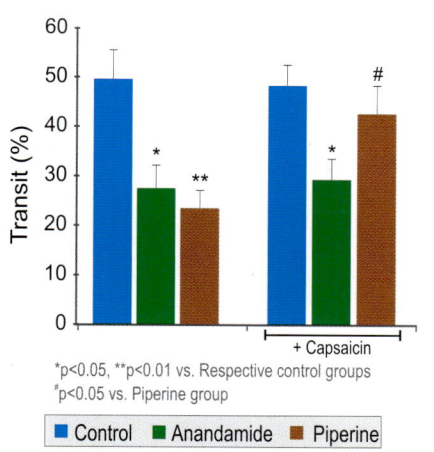

Fig. 59: Effect of piperine on gastrointestinal transit in mice.

It can roughly be correlated that the influence of dietary piperine on food transit time is linked to its beneficial influence either on digestive enzymes or on bile secretion as discussed earlier (Platel and Srinivasan, 2004). Hence, it was hypothesized that digestive stimulant action of piperine is by virtue of accelerated digestive process due to higher availability of digestive enzymes and secretion of bile acids, at the same level of consumption.

Clinical Study

In a pilot study involving 16 healthy volunteers, effect of black pepper on intestinal peristalsis was investigated. Subjects underwent lactulose hydrogen breath test for measuring orocecal transit time on different days with or without capsules containing black pepper (1.5 g). Results suggested that baseline orocecal transit time was increased at the end of the study (90 ± 51 min. vs. 122 ± 88 min., p=0.09). Hence, it was concluded that spices could play an important role in managing various gastrointestinal-related conditions (Vazquez-Olivencia *et al.*, 1992).

C. Influence on Absorptive Function

In vitro Study

An experiment was carried out to understand the influence of piperine on membrane dynamics and permeability characteristics. Results from membrane fluidity studies showed that piperine increased intestinal brush border membrane fluidity. Piperine also stimulated leucine amino peptidase and glycyl-glycine dipeptidase activity by altering enzyme conformation. In conclusion, it was proposed that bioavailability enhancement property of piperine could be attributed to improved absorption, which may be due to altered membrane dynamics and permeability—resulting in improved absorptive surface of small intestine, and this in turn leading to efficient permeation through the epithelial barrier (Khajuria *et al.*, 2002).

Chapter 4
PIPERINE AND ITS HEALTH BENEFITS

Respiratory Health Support

Nearly all of us—be it a child or an elderly person, would have had experienced respiratory health problems in one form or the other, at least once in our lifetime. Respiratory disease is a broad term used to describe different conditions which affect health of the respiratory system. Some of the common conditions that result due to poor lung and respiratory health include mild and self-limiting common cold, other acute infections like upper and lower respiratory tract infections, asthma, sinusitis and allergic rhinitis.

As more and more people are getting exposed to environmental toxins and other irritants in today's industrialized world, one can understand the problem associated with unhealthy respiratory system.

Although substantial understanding in terms of etiology and related immunological factors that lead to respiratory/airway disorders has been made in recent past, current therapeutic options and treatments to address respiratory conditions are not satisfactory. However, traditional knowledge base, which has been documented throughout recorded history and validated by the modern research, is considered to be effective therapeutic alternative or as complementary treatment choice that can augment existing therapies (Rogerio et al., 2016).

Hence, herbal medicine and/or bioactive natural products, such as piperine are believed to have the potential to support lung and respiratory health due to their well-documented health benefits, including relief from respiratory infections, asthma, cough and common cold, immune stimulating effects and clearing airway congestion (Rehman et al., 2015).

Chapter 4
PIPERINE AND ITS HEALTH BENEFITS

In vitro Study

A set of *in vitro* experiments were carried out by Rehman *et al.* to determine potential bronchodilatory effects of crude extract and various fractions of black pepper (i.e. aqueous, chloroform, ethyl acetate and petroleum ether) and pure piperine using tracheal tissues. In one experiment, isolated guinea-pig tracheal preparations were used to detect bronchodilator effects against carbachol and K^+ (80 mM) induced sustained contractions in tracheal ring preparations. Additionally, isoprenaline concentration-response curves (CRCs) were also constructed to evaluate effect of test extracts or standard drugs on smooth muscle relaxation. In another experiment, effects of test extracts and drugs on spontaneous beating of atria, which were isolated from guinea-pigs, were studied.

Results revealed that both crude extract of black pepper and piperine showing similar pattern of inhibition against carbachol- and K^+ (80 mM) induced contractions in guinea-pig tracheal preparations in a concentration-dependent manner (Fig. 60A and 60B), while potentiated isoprenaline CRCs and suppressed Ca^{2+} CRCs.

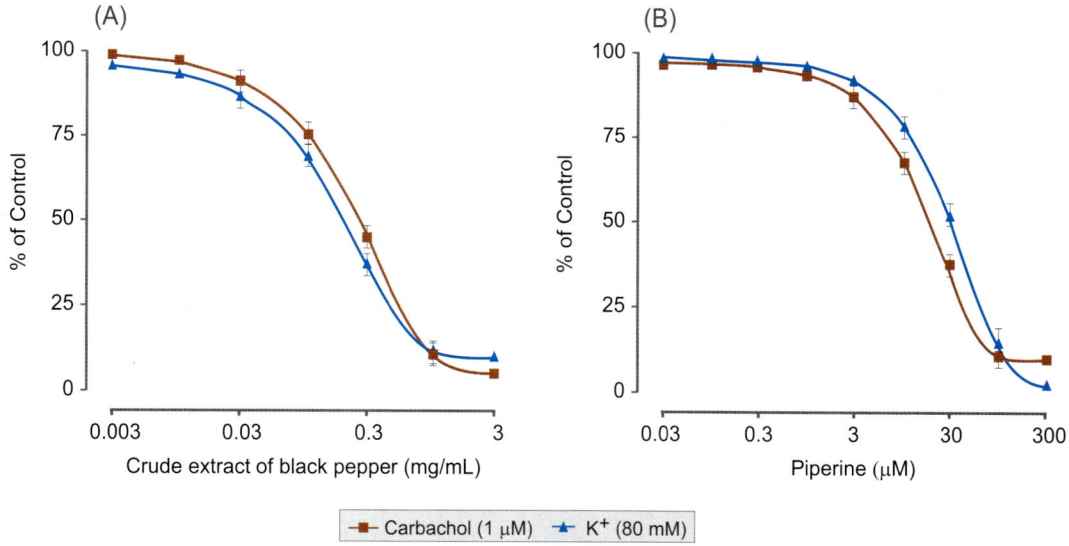

Fig. 60: Inhibitory effects of (A) Crude extract of black pepper (B) Piperine against carbachol- and K^+-induced contraction in isolated guinea-pig tracheal preparations.

In guinea-pig atrial preparations, both crude extract of black pepper and piperine showed stimulatory and inhibitory effects on rate and force of contraction. Various fractions of black pepper extract showed similar activities with varied potency in both the experiments.

In conclusion, black pepper extract and piperine possess bronchodilatory effects due to their ability to inhibit phosphodiesterase enzyme activity and block Ca^{2+} channels, thus may be useful nutraceuticals or functional food ingredients to treat asthma and other airway diseases (Rehman et al., 2015).

In vivo Studies

In an *in vivo* experiment, protective role of piperine against ovalbumin-induced allergic rhinitis was evaluated by Aswar *et al*. Swiss albino mice were sensitized with 500 µl sensitization solution (comprising of 50 mg ovalbumin, 1000 mg aluminium hydroxide and 0.5 ml of 1x1010 *Bordetella bronchiseptica*, a respiratory pathogen) on day 1, 3, 5, 7, 9, 11 and 13 via i.p. injection, except normal (vehicle) animals. Remaining animals that were administered sensitization solution were further divided into different treatment groups and treated with piperine (10, 20 and 40 mg/kg; p.o.) or montelukast (10 mg/kg; p.o.), a standard drug, from day 14 to day 20.

On day 21, all animals were again challenged with 0.5 µl of sensitization solution intranasally, and were evaluated for various physiological (i.e. sneezing, nasal rubbing and nasal redness), biochemical (i.e. estimation of nitric oxide and histamine concentration, and measurement of serum levels of IL-6, IL-1β and IgE) parameters, and spleen weight. Histopathological evaluation (i.e. nasal mucosa, lungs and spleen) was also performed.

Evaluation of physiological parameters suggested that treatment with piperine dose-dependently decreased sneezing and nasal rubbing significantly ($p<0.001$), and effects were comparable to that of montelukast, the standard. Nasal redness was also attenuated significantly by piperine (Table 20).

Group	Treatment	Sneezing/unit time	Nasal rubbing/unit time	Nasal redness
I	Normal	15.83 ± 1.86	19.33 ± 1.44	0.66 ± 0.21
II	Allergic Rhinitis control	79.17 ± 3.17###	71.67 ± 3.29###	2.66 ± 0.21#
III	Montelukast (10 mg/kg)	29.50 ± 2.99***	29.83 ± 1.92***	1.50 ± 0.42
IV	Piperine (10 mg/kg)	29.83 ± 1.24***	29.00 ± 2.25***	1.50 ± 0.22
V	Piperine (20 mg/kg)	26.27 ± 2.82***	23.83 ± 1.83***	1.83 ± 0.40
VI	Piperine (40 mg/kg)	17.83 ± 1.66***	19.67 ± 1.11***	1.33 ± 0.21

Values are mean ± SEM; #$p<0.05$, ###$p<0.001$ vs. Normal control group; ***$p<0.001$ vs Allergic rhinitis control group

Table 20: Protective role of piperine treatment on physiological parameters in ovalbumin-induced allergic rhinitis.

Data from biochemical parameters evaluation showed that piperine treatment ameliorated allergic and inflammatory mediators. A marked increase ($p<0.001$) in the levels of nitric oxide (a mediator in regulating patency of airways), histamine (a known agent for manifestation of certain allergic reactions) as well as other important inflammatory mediators like IL-6, IL-1β and IgE was observed in the allergic rhinitis control group when compared to normal control group. However, treatment with piperine was able to reduce these levels in a dose-dependent manner.

Sensitization with ovalbumin containing solution led to significantly enlarged spleen (characteristic feature of infection or immune response) in allergic rhinitis control group. In groups treated with piperine significant decrease in the spleen weight ($p<0.001$) was observed. Similar results were observed when histopathological evaluation was carried out. Treatment with ovalbumin resulted in degeneration and inflammation in nasal mucosa, lungs and spleen tissues, whereas piperine-treatment was found to exhibit protection against alterations in all 3 tissues in a dose-dependent way.

Overall, it was concluded that piperine was able to prevent allergic responses via mast cell-stabilizing activity, as confirmed by the data from mast cell degranulation experiment, and hence provides protection against ovalbumin-induced allergic rhinitis (Aswar *et al.*, 2015).

Another study was carried by Rehman *et al.* to investigate the potential effect of crude extract and various fractions of black pepper (i.e. aqueous, chloroform, ethyl acetate and petroleum ether) and pure piperine to induce bronchodilator effects in anesthetized rats.

In anesthetized SD rats, bronchoconstriction was induced by administering carbachol (100 µg/kg) and changes in airway resistance were recorded by using a pressure transducer. Bronchodilator effects of test extracts and standard drugs were evaluated by administering them intravenously 5 min. prior to carbachol treatment. Changes in airway resistance were measured again and compared with baseline readings.

The experiment results demonstrated that crude extract and different fractions of black pepper and piperine were able to relieve carbachol-induced bronchospasm in a dose-dependent manner (Fig. 61A and 61B).

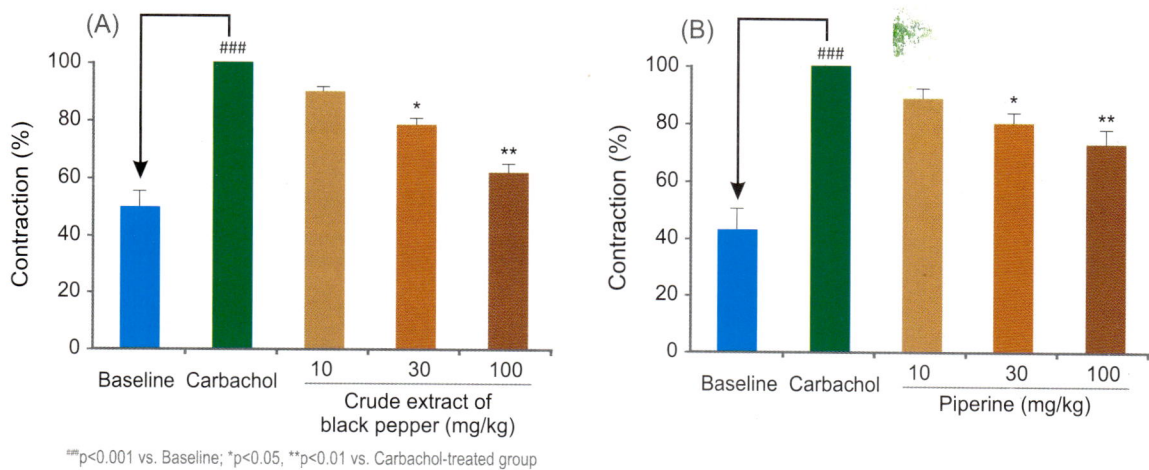

$^{\#\#\#}p<0.001$ vs. Baseline; $^{*}p<0.05$, $^{**}p<0.01$ vs. Carbachol-treated group

Fig. 61: Bronchodilator effects of (A) Crude extract of black pepper (B) Piperine in anesthesized rats

The data emphasized on the potential benefits of black pepper extract and piperine in treating airway disorders, such as bronchitis and asthma (Rehman et al., 2015).

Protective role of piperine against LPS-induced acute lung injury and underlying anti-inflammatory mechanism was evaluated *in vivo* by Lu *et al.* In the present study, 1 h post LPS challenge, mice were treated with different doses of piperine (15, 30 and 60 mg/kg; i.p.). After 12 h of LPS administration, mice were euthanized to collect bronchoalveolar lavage fluid (BALF) and lung tissues for further analysis. Furthermore, parameters like histological examination, lung wet/dry ratio, myeloperoxidase activity (to assess neutrophil accumulation in lung tissues) and levels of inflammatory cytokines (e.g. TNF-α, IL-6, IL-1β) in BALF, and Western blot analysis for analysing NF-κB activation were carried out.

Histological analysis showed that piperine treatment was able to attenuate the severity of lung injuries induced by LPS. Lung wet/dry ratio (a measure to assess the edema of the lung)

Chapter 4
PIPERINE AND ITS HEALTH BENEFITS

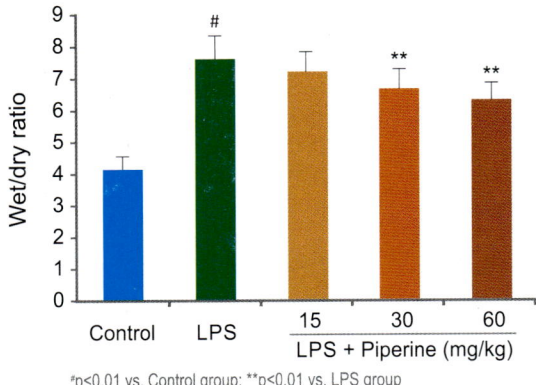

Fig. 62: Protective effect of piperine against LPS-induced lung edema.

also revealed that LPS challenge resulted in significant increase in the lung edema, which was decreased upon piperine treatment (Fig. 62). Similar results were obtained from myeloperoxidase assay and inflammatory cytokines level measurement, wherein a dose-dependent efficacy of piperine was seen in inhibiting LPS-induced myeloperoxidase activity and production of inflammatory cytokines.

Data from the Western blot analysis demonstrated that LPS induced the significant activation of NF-κB and IκBα degradation in lung tissues, which was effectively inhibited by piperine in a dose-dependent manner.

Overall, it was concluded that modulation of NF-κB signaling pathways could be the underlying mechanism by which piperine ameliorates LPS-induced acute lung injury (Lu et al., 2016).

Chapter 4
PIPERINE AND ITS HEALTH BENEFITS

Ergogenic Effects

In today's world of sports, influence of nutrition on training and/or competition performance is gaining interest. Modern training programs also understand the importance of nutrition in sports. Consequently, sports nutrition is believed to be one of the most important segments of sports science. Today, modern day athletes need simple, practical and achievable dietary advice to reach their physical goals and out-perform their competitors. Hence, worldwide, a large percentage of athletes/ sports personnel are using dietary supplements (Williams, 2004).

According to the Dietary Supplement Health and Education Act (DSHEA), United States, dietary supplements are the food (and not drugs), and are substances added to the diet, and may include vitamins, minerals, amino acids, herbs or botanicals and metabolites/ constituents/extracts or combination of any of these ingredients (Williams, 2004).

Phytonutrients derived from various plant foods or herbs form popular dietary supplements. Athletes as well as other fitness enthusiasts are also known to be benefitted from such supplements, in terms of improved physiological or metabolic responses that may enhance exercise performance or overall endurance (Williams, 2006).

Various phytochemicals, including piperine have been commonly used as thermogenic aids to improve metabolism and performance (Walter et al., 2009). In addition, given the fact that piperine is a naturally available thermonutrient and bioenhancer, it could play an important role in improving the endurance of not only the hard-core athletes but also of the people willing to maintain healthy lifestyle.

Piperine Helps Improve Absorption of Branched Chain Amino Acids

Amino acids are known to have ergogenic effects in athletes and physically-active individuals by influencing their endurance and performance in several ways. Branched chain amino acids (i.e. leucine, isoleucine and valine), the essential amino acids, which constitute approximately one-third of skeletal muscle protein play an important role in stimulating protein synthesis and energy production. It has been shown that BCAAs enhance performance in endurance exercise by modifying fuel use, protecting body from adverse effects of overtraining and by delaying mental fatigue (Williams, 2005; Ohtani *et al.*, 2006).

Furthermore, research also suggests that apart from performance benefits during aerobic-based exercise, BCAAs may also help in improving mental performance.

In vitro Study

Piperine's effect on bioavailability enhancement of amino acids was evaluated by Johri *et al*. In this *in vitro* experiment, treating freshly isolated epithelial cells from rat jejunum with piperine enhanced the uptake of 3 radiolabelled BCAAs (i.e. L-leucine, L-isoleucine and L-valine) significantly (Table 9) in an identical manner (Johri *et al.*, 1992). Hence, co-administration of piperine with BCAAs would further improve absorption of BCAAs, which in turn helps enhance endurance and performance of sports personnel.

Chapter 4
PIPERINE AND ITS HEALTH BENEFITS

Co-supplementaion of Resveratrol and BioPerine® Improves Adaptations to Low-intensity Stimuli

Clinical Study

In a double-blind, placebo-controlled, 4-week clinical trial, 16 healthy young adults (nine males and seven females) were evaluated for the influence of co-supplementation of resveratrol with BioPerine® on muscle mitochondrial function with sub-maximal endurance training.

Participants were supervised to undergo a 30 min. exercise training procedure, involving forearm wrist flexor exercises of the non-dominant arm for 3 times per week over 4 weeks. The dominant arm was not trained and used as the untrained control arm for each subject. Participants were randomly assigned (n=8) to receive 2 pills every morning, each containing resveratrol (500 mg) and BioPerine® (10 mg); or 2 identically appearing placebo pills containing flour.

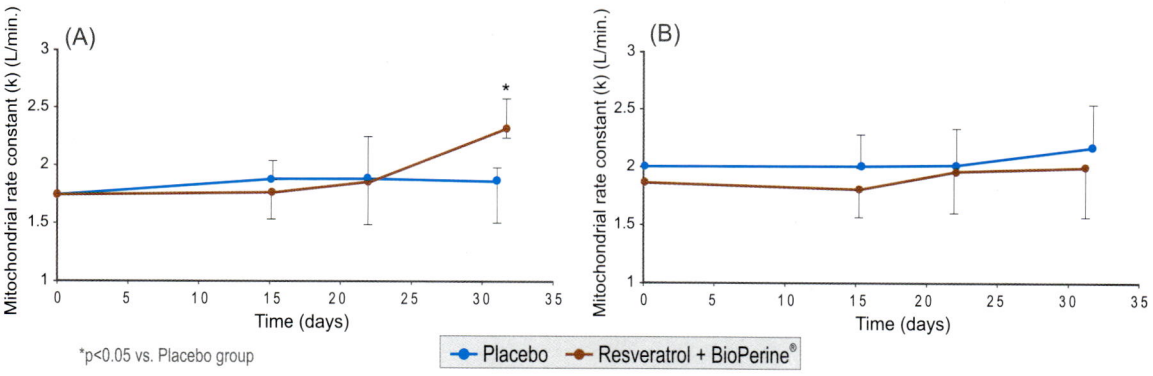

Fig. 63: Effect of resveratrol and BioPerine® combination on muscle oxidative capacity in (A) Trained arm (B) Untrained arm.

Mitochondrial function was evaluated with short bout of voluntary exercise to increase metabolic rate; after the exercise the rate of recovery of metabolic rate was measured.

The mitochondrial measurements were recorded using near infrared spectroscopy for 45 min. on week 0, 2, 3 and 4. At the end of the trial, results demonstrated that trained arm in active group showed a significant recovery of muscle oxidative capacity (measured in terms of average mitochondrial rate constant, k) compared to placebo group (Fig. 63A). However, there was no difference between untrained arm in active and placebo group (Fig. 63B).

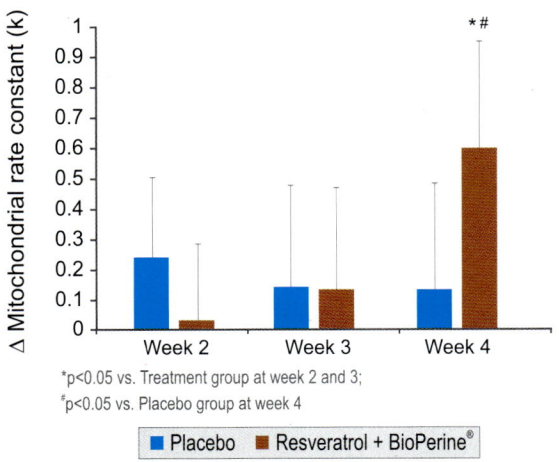

Fig. 64: Effect of resveratrol and BioPerine® combination on change in mitochondrial function (ANCOVA model).

Similarly, in ANCOVA model of analysis, a significant difference in the change in mitochondrial function from baseline to post-testing between the active-trained arm and the placebo-trained arm ($p=0.02$) was observed, with the treatment group increasing about 40% from the baseline ($\Delta k=0.58$), while the placebo group increased about 10% from the baseline (Fig. 64). However, no significant difference was observed between treated-untrained arm and placebo-untrained arm.

Overall, given the fact that choice of low-intensity stimulus in current study, authors concluded that co-supplementation of resveratrol and BioPerine® could be significant for the general population, especially who may be unable to perform high-intensity exercise (Polley *et al.*, 2016).

Curcumin and Piperine Supplementation Attenuates Exercise-induced Muscle Damage

Clinical Findings

Recently, in a randomized, balanced, cross-over design study, effects of supplementation of curcumin and piperine combination on the recovery kinetics following exercise-induced muscle damage were evaluated in 10 elite level rugby players.

This study was divided into two phases (each of 4 days duration), separated by 15 days. During the first phase, participants were divided into 4 groups (i.e. Dominant leg–curcumin+piperine, Non-dominant leg– curcumin+piperine, Dominat leg– placebo, Non-dominat leg– placebo) and were asked to consume curcumin (2 g) and piperine (20 mg) supplement or placebo thrice a day during 4-day experimental condition (i.e. 48 h of pre-exercise and 48 h post-exercise).

The ratio of curcumin (2 g) and piperine (20 mg) combination was believed to enable the increased bioavailability of curcumin as per Shoba *et al*. (1998). During pre-exercise duration supplement was divided into 3 doses (scheduled for every 6 h), however, based on the

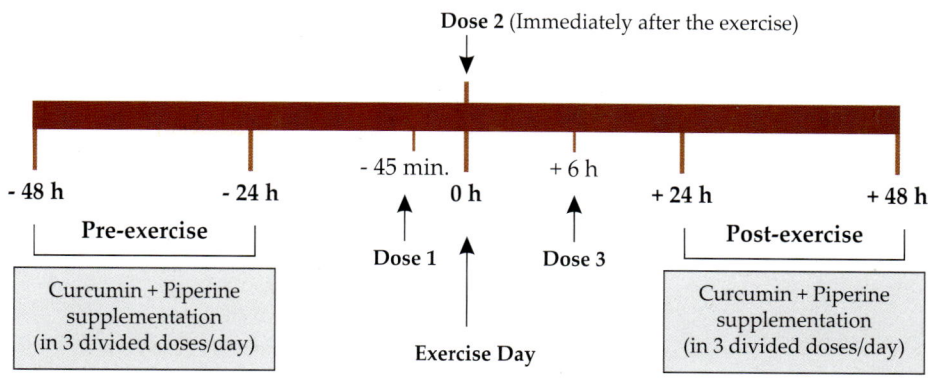

Fig. 65: Protocol describing curcumin and piperine supplementation during the experiment.

observations by Shoba *et al*. (1998) suggesting that bioavailability of curcumin reaches its peak 45 min. after consumption in the presence of piperine, on the exercise day the first intake was set to be 45 min. prior to the exercise. And the second dose was provided immediately after the exercise, while the last dose was given 6 h after the second dose (Fig. 65).

Similar protocol was followed for the second session, but participants were evaluated on the other leg and in other condition as that of the first session. During both sessions, participants were evaluated for baseline testing followed by the exercise task on the first day, and immediately after the exercise task, and then 24 h, 48 h and 72 h post-exercise.

Different parameters were used to assess the muscle function apart from evaluating total blood creatine kinase concentration and general muscle soreness and specific quadriceps level of soreness in participants.

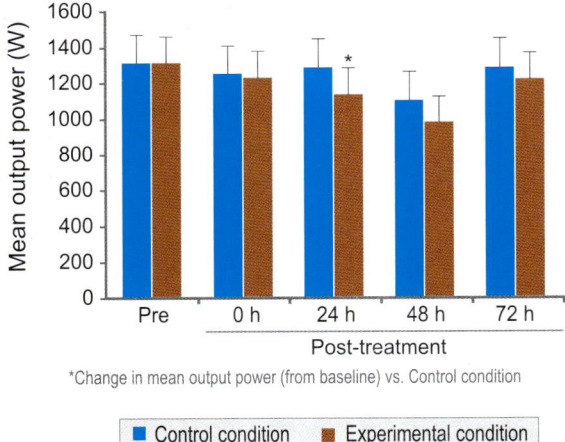

Fig. 66: Effect of supplementation of curcumin and piperine combination on the mean power output during 6s sprint.

Results showed that selected exercise task was able to induce muscle damage as indicated by reduced muscle function (considered as a marker to muscle damage) as well as elevated muscle soreness up to 48 h post-exercise and elevated levels of creatine kinase up to 72 h after the exercise in the control condition. However, in experimental condition, supplementation with curcumin and piperine combination was able to moderately lower the sprint mean power output (from baseline) 24 h post-exercise in comparison to control condition treated with placebo (Fig. 66).

Hence, authors concluded that supplementation with piperine combination pre- and post-exercise session can help recover from some aspects of the muscle damage (Delecroix *et al*., 2017).

Other Potential Benifits of Piperine on Exercise-associated Implications

Protection against Exercise-induced Oxidative Stress and Inflammatory Response

Physical training/exercise could lead to biochemical adaptive response and thus can be regarded as a prototype of physical stress, as several physical stressors, such as surgery, trauma, burn, sepsis are known to induce a pattern of hormonal and immunological responses, which is something similar to that induced by exercise (Pedersen, 2000).

Production of free radicals (e.g. ROS) during aerobic cellular metabolism (e.g. during high-intensity exercise or sports activity) is believed to modulate signaling processes as key regulatory mediators—thus leading to muscle damage and/or impaired muscle function (Peternelj and Coombes, 2011; Pingitore et al., 2015).

As far as the relationship between exercise and oxidative stress is concerned, it varies depending on the mode, intensity and duration of exercise. For example, regular low or moderate training is believed to be beneficial, whereas intense, non-usual and eccentric muscle exercise has been found to initiate production of various pro-inflammatory mediators—a local response to tissue injury, which could further result in skeletal muscle damage (Pingitore et al., 2015; Pedersen, 2000).

In recent times, a lot of attention has been paid to understand the role of antioxidant supplements in supporting endogenous defence systems. It has been studied that antioxidant supplementation helps attenuate or minimize exercise-induced oxidative stress, reduce muscle damage and improve the performance (Peternelj and Coombes, 2011; Pingitore et al., 2015).

Chapter 4
PIPERINE AND ITS HEALTH BENEFITS

So, ingredients like piperine, owing to their proven antioxidant and anti-inflammatory potential as expatiated earlier in this section could prove effective in providing optimal protection against exercise-related oxidative stress and decreased muscle function and/or damage. However, more research is warranted to further prove potential benefits of piperine in this regard.

Importance of Reflexes, Reaction Time and Mental Performance in Sports: Potential Role of Piperine

An athlete should be able to make good coordination between reflexes, reaction time, think faster and make decisions—in general; he/she should be multitasking whilst in the midst of high-performance sporting competition. Thus, for a player it is imperative to have optimal balance, proprioception and cognition—different aspects of the brain's ability to perform at this high level whilst efficiently coordinating the speed, power and endurance.

These are the vital skills that determine player's success during athletic participation. Most of athletes are now interested to learn what is necessary to do well cognitively in their sport and perform well.

Given the fact that piperine is known for its beneficial role in promoting brain health and neuropharmacological activities, consumption of piperine would also satisfy the cognitive needs of an athlete very well, as evident from several study findings (discussed earlier in this section). However, further studies involving different sports personals/physically active individuals are advised in order to ascertain its merits in sports set up.

In conclusion, black pepper, an Indian native spice, has been cherished for several thousands of years because of its characteristic principles—attributed to the alkaloid piperine. In recent decades, a number of independent investigators have reported black pepper extract or its bioactive compound piperine to possess varied health benefits as well as several physiological effects. The most far-reaching attributes include enhancing the bioavailability of phytochemicals and other xenobiotics, stimulation of digestive enzymes as well as many potential therapeutic applications ranging from anti-inflammatory effects, management of metabolic disorders, neuropharmacological benefits to anticarcinogenic potential to ergogenic effects and respiratory health support, as proven by several *in vitro*, *in vivo* and clinical studies.

Moreover, apart from the molecular basis for the pharmacological properties of black pepper extract and piperine against various disease conditions, modern science has paid significant attention to the metabolism and safety of black pepper extract as well, which will be discussed in the following sections in detail.

Chapter 5
Metabolism of Piperine

Understanding the biological fate of piperine, a highly lipophilic and bitter molecule, once it enters our body system is essential, considering its wide spectrum of physiological effects and pharmacological actions as well as its omnipresence in the form of dietary ingredient.

Very few studies have been carried out to determine pharmacokinetics, particularly, metabolism and excretion of piperine. In 1986, Bhat and Chandrasekhara demonstrated that 97% of piperine was absorbed when administered to male albino rats at a dose of 170 mg/kg (p.o.) or 85 mg/kg (i.p.), irrespective of the mode of dosing. Remaining 3% was detected in the feces, while it was not detectable in urine.

Moreover, about 47–64% of the added piperine (200–1000 µg) in the everted sacs of rat intestine disappeared from the mucosal side. Absorbed piperine could be traced in both the serosal fluid and in the intestinal tissue—indicating that piperine did not undergo any metabolic change during the process of absorption.

Additionally, highest concentration of piperine in the stomach and small intestine was found to be attained at about 6 h. In serum, kidney and spleen only traces (<0.15%) of piperine were detected from 30 min. to 24 h, while about 1–2.5% of the intraperitoneally and 0.1–0.25% of the orally administered dose of piperine was detected in the liver 0.5–6 h after administration (Bhat and Chandrasekhara, 1986a).

Chapter 5
METABOLISM OF PIPERINE

Similar observations were made by Suresh and Srinivasan when they studied *in vitro* absorption of piperine in rat intestines. When everted sacs of rat intestines were incubated with 50–1000 μg of piperine, about 44–63% of piperine disappeared from the mucosal side with maximum absorption (i.e. 63%) at 800 μg concentration. When piperine was associated with mixed micelles, its *in vitro* absorption was relatively higher (Suresh and Srinivasan, 2007a).

Overall, it was concluded that scission of the methylenedioxy group of piperine, glucuronidation and sulphation were the major steps in the metabolism of piperine in rats since conjugated uronic acids, sulphates and phenols were higher in excretion (Bhat and Chandrasekhara, 1986a).

Further detailed metabolic disposition of piperine, following biotransformation pathway of piperine in rats was proposed by Bhat and Chandrasekhara in 1987. This study involved determination of urinary and biliary metabolites of piperine using thin-layer chromatography, high-performance liquid chromatography (HPLC) and combined gas chromatography-mass spectrometry. From the experiments, it was observed that piperine was extensively metabolized, giving rise to several metabolites, of which 5 were identified (Fig. 67A).

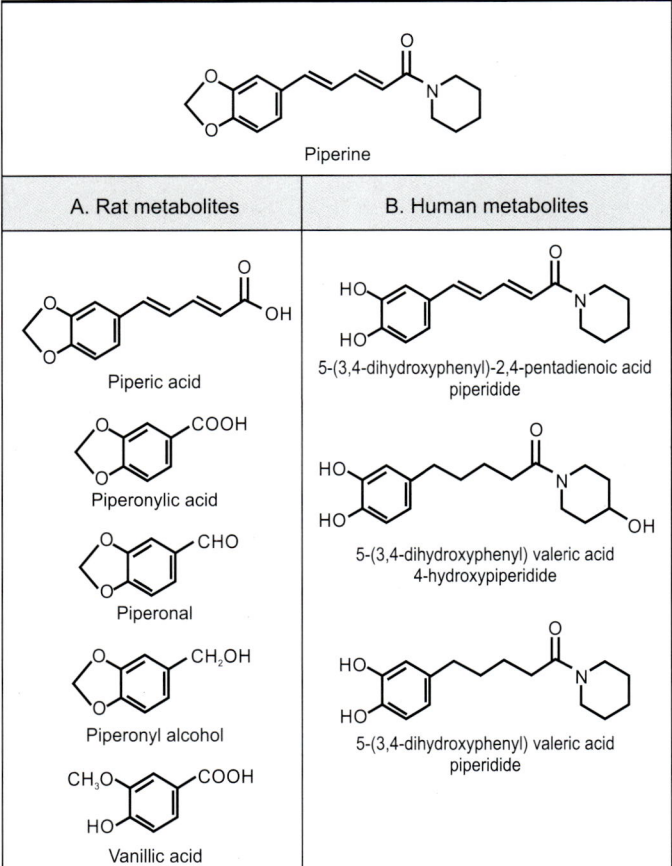

Fig. 67: Metabolites of piperine in (A) Rats (B) Humans.
(Reproduced from Bajad *et al.* 2003)

Chapter 5
METABOLISM OF PIPERINE

Four metabolites of piperine, viz. piperonylic acid, piperonal, piperonyl alcohol and vanillic acid were detected in the free form in 0–96 h urine samples, whereas only piperic acid, the fifth metabolite, was identified in 0–6 h bile samples. It was believed that metabolism of piperine would involve amidase enzyme, which reportedly converts piperine to piperic acid, which in turn gets metabolized to piperonal, piperonylic acid and vanillic acid, and their metabolites (Fig. 68). In this study, other principal route of piperine metabolism was hypothesized to be through cleavage of the methylenedioxy group. Catechols, the major metabolites, are then O-methylated to methoxyphenols, of which only vanillic acid was identified in the current experiment. Alternatively, vanillic acid might have also arisen from the oxidation of the intermediate aldehyde vanillin (Bhat and Chandrasekhara, 1987b).

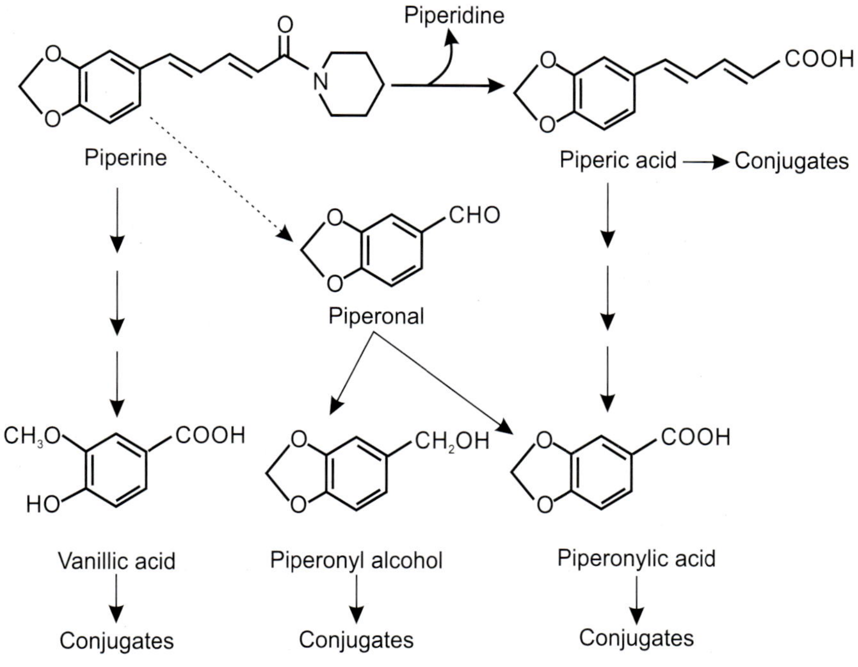

Fig. 68: Proposed biotransformation pathway of piperine in rats.
(Reproduced from Bhat and Chandrasekhara, 1987b)

Although no systematic studies have been carried out so far in humans, Claus and Gerhard accidently found three urinary metabolites of piperine in athletes, which were entirely

Chapter 5
METABOLISM OF PIPERINE

different from those reported in rats by Bhat and Chandrasekhara (1987b) (Fig. 67B). Here, after several days of oral intake of piperine (25 mg), urinary metabolites like 5-(3,4-dihydroxyphenyl) valeric acid piperidide (1.49 mg) and 5-(3,4-dihydroxyphenyl) valeric acid 4-hydroxypiperidide (hydroxylated at position 4 of the piperidide ring) (0.64 mg) were recovered from most of the volunteers. However, these metabolites could not be detected in about 15% of the volunteers, instead 5-(3,4-dihydroxyphenyl)-2,4-pentadienoic acid piperidide, the third metabolite, was traced in their urine samples (Claus and Gerhard, 1984).

During an attempt to further study the reported differences in metabolism of piperine in rats and humans, Bajad *et al.* detected a new major urinary metabolite, characterized as 5-(3,4-methylenedioxy phenyl)-2,4-pentadienoic acid-N-(3-yl propionic acid)-amide in rat urine and plasma. This metabolite has a unique structure in that it retains the methylenedioxy ring and conjugated double bonds, while the piperidine ring is modified to form the propionic acid group. Since no metabolites were detected in feces, it was suggested that kidney is the major route of excretion for piperine metabolites in rats (Bajad et al., 2003).

To understand the oral absorption dynamics of piperine in intestine, cycloheximide treatment, and exclusion of Na^+ salts from incubating medium were used as variables in an intestinal everted sac model. Various parameters like absorption $t_{1/2}$, absorption rate, clearance and apparent permeability coefficient were computed using this model. The data suggested that faster absorption of piperine across the intestinal barrier could possibly be due to its apolar nature, which is responsible for apolar complex formation with xenobiotics and solutes. It has been thought to modulate membrane dynamics due to its easy partitioning, thus helping in efficient permeability across the barrier (Khajuria et al., 1998b).

Piperine, being essentially water-insoluble, is thought to be assisted by serum albumin for its transport in blood once it gets absorbed by the intestine. Hence, a study was carried out to examine binding of piperine to serum albumin using steady-state and time-resolved fluorescence techniques. Binding constant for the interaction of piperine with human serum albumin, which was invariant with temperature in the range of 17–47 °C, was found to be

0.5×10^5 M^{-1} having stoichiometry of 1:1. Results indicated binding of piperine to the subdomain-IB of serum albumin. Thus, these observations will be useful in understanding the transport of piperine in blood under physiological conditions (Suresh *et al.*, 2007b).

Chapter 6
Long-term Safety of Piperine

An increasing global awareness on "what we eat makes us what we are" has led to the popularity of botanicals and herbs as natural food and dietary supplements. As a result, a number of plant-derived products have become an integral part of human diet.

Although the use of nature-derived botanicals and dietary supplements as an adjunct to improve quality of life or for their purported medical benefits has become increasingly common, only a few natural products have been subjected to toxicological and nutritional assessment. The basic reasons could be the fact that they are traditionally regarded as safe to consume, absence of evidence of harm and because of their long history of use. However, reassurance about the safety of such products is very essential in the modern world to provide greater confidence to the customers. Hence, all the traditional understanding and well documented long history of safe use could form a bench mark for the comparative safety assessment of newer natural products.

Safety results from animal studies and observations from human exposure (i.e. assessment of safety for a food or dietary ingredient to determine safe level of ingestion compared to the estimated daily intake from its proposed uses) play an important role in ascertaining safe consumption of natural compounds. A regulatory framework for herbal medicines, in addition to safety guarantee system comprising

Chapter 6
LONG-TERM SAFETY OF PIPERINE

rational clinical practice and risk monitoring can provide greater assurance to consumers in terms of improved safety of phytoextracts, and their role in maintaining overall well being.

Black pepper, in addition to its use as a spice in foodstuff and its preservative properties, has also been used as an additive for animal nutrition. Ayurveda has descriptions about the use of black pepper for a wide variety of health benefits.

Black pepper, the "king of spices", has been in use for a long time and it fetches the highest return among all the spices known, as judged from the volume of international trade (Srinivasan, 2007). In the United States, black pepper is officially classified as "**Generally Recognized As Safe**" **(GRAS)** substance as a source of essential oils, oleoresins and natural extractives for general use in foods under 21 CFR 182.20. The GRAS approval is accorded to such items which demonstrate safety of long-term use or traditional use in food (Code of Federal Regulations, 2016).

According to Kindell (1984), the average daily consumption of black pepper in the United States was 359 mg per person in 1978. Given that the content of piperine in black pepper varies between 5–9%, this would suggest a daily per capita consumption of approximately 18.0–32.3 mg of piperine (Table 21) (Kindell, 1984; Bhardwaj et al., 2002).

Over the period of time, there has been a considerable increase in the consumption of black pepper. As per the import data for the year 2007, around 31,000 tons of ground pepper has been imported by the United States alone (of which 7,760 tons came from three countries: India, Brazil and Vietnam) (Anonymous, 2007). Hence, based on these import data one can presume that import of black pepper by the United States and in turn the per capita consumption has significantly gone up since 1970s.

	mg/person	mg/kg*
Black pepper	359	6.0
Piperine	18.0–32.3	0.3–0.54

*Average human weight estimated at 60 kg

Table 21: Estimated average human consumption of black pepper/piperine.

Chapter 6
LONG-TERM SAFETY OF PIPERINE

In other words, millions of people in the United States have consumed piperine over a period of 35 years or so, and during this period no serious adverse effects have been reported in relation to chronic consumption of piperine in the range 18.0–32.3 mg/day. Overall, this data serves as sufficient and excellent evidence assuring the long-term safety of piperine.

However, large consumption of black pepper by the population of the United States led to question the potential biological effects of piperine, as few controversial reports cited safety concerns of black pepper or piperine as a food additive (Kindell, 1984).

A few researchers had raised concerns over the presence of chemical constituents like safrole in black pepper for their possible carcinogenic properties or as co-carcinogens or tumor promotion (Majeed et al., 1999). However, studies have suggested that piperine is not implicated as a possible tumorigenic or carcinogenic compound (Concon et al., 1979; Majeed et al., 1999). Also safrole is not detected in BioPerine® preparations.

In addition, several experimental studies support the safety-in-use of black pepper and its preparations. These studies did not show any adverse effects of black pepper or its preparations at the commonly used levels.

Chapter 6
LONG-TERM SAFETY OF PIPERINE

Acute and Sub-acute Studies

In an acute toxicity study, the median lethal dose (LD_{50}) of piperine for a single intravenous, intraperitoneal, subcutaneous, intragastric and intramuscular in adult male mice were 15.1, 43, 200, 330 and 400 mg/kg, respectively. Compared to the adult male mice, the intraperitoneal LD_{50} value was higher in adult female (60 mg/kg) and in weanling male mice (132 mg/kg). In adult female rats, the intraperitoneal LD_{50} value was 33.5 mg/kg, whereas the intragastric LD_{50} value was increased to 514 mg/kg (Piyachaturawat et al., 1983).

In a sub-acute toxicity study, adult female rats were given piperine at a dose of 100, 250, 350 or 500 mg/kg for 7 consecutive days. A dose-related decrease in body weight gain was noted. Although no deaths occurred at the lower doses, a slight reduction in the body weight gain was reported at 250 mg/kg. Histological examination showed changes in the stomach, urinary bladder, adrenal glands and small intestine. Mild fatty infiltration in the liver and cell necrosis in the corpora lutea were the other significant histopathological changes reported (Piyachaturawat et al., 1983).

However, other studies showed no adverse effect in rats fed with higher dose of black pepper or piperine, as indicated by growth, organ weight and levels of blood constituents (Srinivasan and Satyanarayana, 1981).

Sub-chronic Study

In continuation to earlier observations (Srinivasan and Satyanarayana, 1981), long-term effects of black pepper, its oleoresin or piperine were investigated by Bhat and Chandrasekhara (1986b).

In a long-term toxicity study, male Wistar rats were fed with diets containing black pepper oleoresin at a concentration of 110, 220 and 440 ppm, pepper at 2000 ppm or piperine at

100 ppm for a period of 8 weeks. Results have shown that ingestion of black pepper, its oleoresin or piperine at doses 5–20 times the average daily human intake did not cause any adverse effect on rats for the following parameters (Bhat and Chandrasekhara, 1986b):

- Growth, food efficiency ratio and organ weights (liver, kidney, spleen and adipose tissue)
- Red blood cells, white blood cells and differential counts
- Levels of blood constituents like hemoglobin, total serum proteins, albumin, globulin, sugar and cholesterol
- Levels of serum aminotransferases and phosphatases
- Fat and nitrogen balance

Immunotoxicity Studies

Dogra *et al.* investigated the immunotoxicological effects of piperine in Swiss male mice at dose levels of 1.12, 2.25 and 4.5 mg/kg for five consecutive days. Results demonstrated that piperine at all dose levels had no overt toxic effects and weight of the liver was found to be normal. Based on the effect of piperine on the functions of spleen, thymus and lymph nodes, the no observed adverse effect level (NOAEL) at 1.12 mg/kg was considered as immunologically safe (Dogra *et al.*, 2004). Piperine has also been shown to be immunoprotective towards cadmium, a well known environmental carcinogen, and could be considered as the drug of choice under immune compromised conditions (Pathak and Khandelwal, 2008).

Genotoxicity Studies

Piperine was found to be non-genotoxic by several studies (Singh *et al.*, 1994; Karekar *et al.*, 1996; Selvendiran *et al.*, 2005c). In Swiss albino mice, it was shown that piperine at six different doses, in the range of 0.005–10 µmol/plate, did not induce his+ revertants, with or without metabolic activation—indicating its non-mutagenic nature in the AMES test using *Salmonella typhimurium* (Karekar *et al.*, 1996).

In an *in vitro* micronucleus test (MNT), piperine reduced the aflatoxin B1-induced formation of micronuclei in a concentration-dependent manner, showing a negative response against rat hepatoma cells H4IIEC3 (Singh *et al.*, 1994).

In addition, several *in vivo* studies at low dose levels of piperine (up to 75 mg/kg) showed negative results for different end points, such as chromosomal aberration, micronucleus induction, induction of DNA strands or dominant lethal mutation (Muralidhara and Narasimhamurthy, 1990; Karekar *et al.*, 1996). In another study, piperine at doses 10 and 50 mg/kg failed to induce mutations in male germ cells of mice as assessed by sperm shape abnormality and dominant lethal tests (Karekar *et al.*, 1996). Furthermore, oral administration of piperine at doses 25, 50 and 75 mg/kg in mice showed a significant suppression (33.9–66.5%) of micronuclei formation induced by BAP and cyclophosphamide. Observations from this study also corroborated the non-genotoxic property of piperine based on the reduction in the micronuclei formation (Selvendiran *et al.*, 2005c).

When high oral doses (up to 800 mg/kg) of piperine were administered to rats, it did not induce increased incidence of chromosomal aberrations. Piperine produced a statistically significant reduction in cyclophosphamide-induced chromosomal aberrations at a dose of 100 mg/kg and thus, shown to have antimutagenic potential (Wongpa *et al.*, 2007). Following table summarizes the mutagenicity-related studies of piperine (Table 22):

Test System	Endpoint	Concentration	Result	Reference
S. typhimurium	Reverse Mutation	0.005–10 µmole/plate	Negative	Karekar et al., 1996
Swiss mice (bone marrow)	Micronuclei	10 or 20 mg/kg	Negative	Karekar et al., 1996
Swiss mice (bone marrow)	Micronuclei	1, 2 or 4 mg/kg	Negative	Muralidhara and Narasimhamurthy, 1990
Swiss mice (bone marrow)	Micronuclei	Up to 75 mg/kg	Negative	Selvendiran et al., 2005c
Swiss mice	Sperm Morphology	10 or 50 mg/kg	Negative	Karekar et al., 1996
Swiss mice	Sperm Morphology	Up to 75 mg/kg	Negative	Daware et al., 2000
Swiss mice	Sperm Morphology	1, 2, or 4 mg/kg	Negative	Muralidhara and Narasimhamurthy, 1990
Swiss mice Mutation	Dominant Lethal	10 or 50 mg/kg	Negative	Karekar et al., 1996
Swiss mice Mutation	Dominant Lethal	4 mg/kg	Negative	Muralidhara and Narasimhamurthy, 1990

Table 22: Mutagenicity-related studies of piperine.

A few of the conflicting results that were published on piperine's genotoxicity are as follows:

- Alcoholic extract of the mature berries of black pepper induced the genotoxic damage in both *in vitro* (human lymphocytes) and *in vivo* (mouse bone marrow cells) systems (Madrigal-Bujaidar et al., 1997)

- Mice when treated with piperine at doses 143.5, 287 or 574 mg/kg showed an increase in the micronucleus frequency in polychromatic erythrocytes, indicating a clastogenic effect (Lu et al., 2009)

Though the genotoxicity of piperine has been investigated by several researchers previously, owing to lack of data on the dose levels covering a range from 'not toxic' to 'as high as possible', information on the genotoxicity of this traditional herb was considered incomplete until recently. In 2014, in an animal study, it was shown that piperine did not cause micronucleus induction up to the maximum tolerated dose levels as per the regulatory guidelines, thus providing conclusive evidence that piperine is not genotoxic (Thiel et al., 2014).

In vitro MNT by Thiel *et al.* in Chinese hamster ovary cells showed absence of genotoxicity by piperine both in the presence and absence of metabolic activation. Absence of metabolic activation was in line with the previous citation by Singh *et al.* (1994). Though piperine was found to be non-genotoxic, presence of metabolic activation was thought to be due to poor solubility of piperine at higher concentrations in the medium, which in turn led to cytotoxicity and cytostasis (Thiel *et al.*, 2014).

In an *in vivo* MNT, piperine was administered by oral gavage for 2 consecutive days to NMRI mice at dose levels of 0, 143.5, 287 and 574 mg/kg (dose selection was based on the study by Lu *et al.*, 2009).

Three extra groups of animals were exposed to either hyperthermic treatment, which were then treated with chlorpromazine (to induce micronucleus in polychromatic erythrocytes) or treated with cyclophosphamide. Results suggested that piperine showed a significant reduction in core body temperature, decrease in white blood cells and spleen weights. In addition, piperine-treated group showed no increase of micronucleus frequencies compared to control animals in contrast to the earlier study results by Lu *et al.* (2009).

Hence, this study negates earlier findings that had concluded that piperine was genotoxic in terms of dose levels.

Technical reason for the discrepancy of the results could be due to susceptibility of two strains: NMRI mice, a strain that has been extensively used as an experimental animal in many fields of general biology, as well as in pharmacology and toxicology (Thiel *et al.*, 2014) compared to use of Kunming mice in the previous study (Lu *et al.*, 2009).

Carcinogenicity-related Studies

Piperine also provided evidence for chemopreventive activity by inhibition or reduction of tumoriogenic responses in animals treated with known carcinogens, such as BAP (Thiel et al., 2014).

The anti-carcinogenic potential of piperine was studied in mice. Animals were treated orally with BAP (50 mg/kg, weekly twice for 4 weeks), piperine + BAP (during initiation), piperine + BAP (post initiation), and piperine alone (50 mg/kg) for 16 weeks. Results showed that supplementation of piperine effectively suppressed BAP-induced lung carcinogenesis in mice by offering protection from protein damage and also by suppressing cell proliferation (Selvendiran et al., 2004b).

Hepatotoxicity-related Studies

In an *in vivo* study, piperine has been reported to potentiate carbon tetrachloride (CCl_4) induced hepatotoxicity at a dosage of 100 mg/kg by increasing lipid peroxidation (Piyachaturawat et al., 1995). Similarly, in an *in vitro* study, piperine potentiated CCl_4-induced hepatotoxicity by interacting with liver cells and increased the activity of NADPH-cytochrome c reductase. The increase in activity is mainly due to its stimulation of NADPH-cytochrome c reductase, which accelerated biotransformation of CCl_4, thereby increasing lipid peroxidation and enhancing hepatotoxicity (Piyachaturawat et al., 1995).

In another study, piperine exerted a significant protection against *tert*-butyl hydroperoxide and CCl_4 hepatotoxicity by reducing lipid peroxidation in both *in vitro* and *in vivo*, leakage of enzymes (i.e. alanine aminotransaminase and alkaline phosphatase) and also by preventing depletion of glutathione and total thiols in the intoxicated mice (Koul and Kapil, 1993).

Chapter 6
LONG-TERM SAFETY OF PIPERINE

Clinical Studies

A clinical study was carried out at St. John's Medical College, Bangalore, to understand the role of BioPerine® in increasing the bioavailability of Curcumin C3 Complex®. BioPerine® was found to increase the bioavailability of Curcumin C3 Complex® with no reported adverse side effects at the tested dosages (Shoba *et al.*, 1998).

In another randomized, cross-over study, researchers at Tufts University School of Medicine, Boston, USA, studied the interaction between BioPerine®-Curcumin C3 Complex® combination and some commonly used drugs (midazolam, flurbiprofen and acetaminophen). It was concluded that though both Curcumin C3 Complex® and BioPerine® are relatively potent inhibitors of liver enzymes involved in drug metabolism the combination does not have the ability to modify substantial disposition of medication, which are dependent on CYP3A, CYP2C9, UGT and SULT pathways—proving the safety of Curcumin C3 Complex® and BioPerine®. Hence, results of the study provided strong evidence in favor of the use of BioPerine® as a bioenhancer, without any adverse drug reactions (Volak *et al.*, 2013).

Incidentally, the dose of piperine, which increased the bioavailability of the nutrients/drugs studied was several times lower than the estimated amount of piperine consumed daily in the diet by an average individual in the United States (Majeed *et al.*, 1999).

Following table summarizes the studies (Table 23), wherein co-administration of BioPerine® has increased the bioavailability of phytonutrients, minerals and vitamins (Majeed and Majeed., 2015; Khonche *et al.*, 2016; Panahi *et al.*, 2016a & b).

Study Title	Dosage
Curcumin downregulates NF-κB and related genes in patients with multiple myeloma: results of a phase I/II study	Curcumin C3 Complex® + BioPerine® (up to 12 g + 10 mg/day)
Improvement of sulphur mustard-induced chronic pruritus, quality of life and antioxidant status by curcumin: results of a randomized double-blind, placebo-controlled trial	Curcumin C3 Complex® + BioPerine® (1000 mg + 10 mg/day)

Chapter 6
LONG-TERM SAFETY OF PIPERINE

Study Title	Dosage
A randomized, controlled trial on the anti-inflammatory effects of curcumin in patients with chronic sulphur mustard-induced cutaneous complication	Curcumin C3 Complex® + BioPerine® (1000 mg + 10 mg/day)
Effects of curcuminoids-piperine combination on systemic oxidative stress, clinical symptoms and quality of life in subjects with chronic pulmonary complications due to sulphur mustard: a randomized controlled trial	Curcumin C3 Complex® + BioPerine® (1500 mg + 15 mg/day)
Short-term curcuminoids supplementation for chronic pulmonary complications due to sulphur mustard intoxication: positive results of a randomized double-blind placebo-controlled trial	Curcumin C3 Complex® + BioPerine® (1500 mg + 15 mg/day)
Curcuminoids treatment for knee osteoarthritis: a randomized double-blind placebo-controlled trial	Curcumin C3 Complex® + BioPerine® (1500 mg + 15 mg/day)
Mitigation of systemic oxidative stress by curcuminoids in osteoarthritis: results of a randomized controlled trial	Curcumin C3 Complex® + BioPerine® (1500 mg +15 mg/day)
Impact of supplementation with curcuminoids on systemic inflammation in patients with knee osteoarthritis: findings from a randomized, double-blind placebo-controlled trial	Curcumin C3 Complex® + BioPerine® (1500 mg +15 mg/day)
Proof of concept of randomized controlled study of Curcumin C3 Complex® as adjunct treatment in schizophrenia: effects of negative and depressive symptoms	Curcumin C3 Complex® + BioPerine® (1 g + 5 mg/day or 4 g + 20 mg/day)
Investigation of the efficacy of adjunctive therapy with bioavailability-boosted curcuminoids in major depressive disorder	Curcumin C3 Complex® + BioPerine® (1000 mg + 10 mg/day)
Effects of supplementation with curcuminoids on dyslipidemia in obese patients: a randomized, crossover trial	Curcumin C3 Complex® + BioPerine® (1000 mg + 10 mg/day)
Curcuminoids modulate pro-oxidant-antioxidant balance but not the immune response to heat shock protein 27 and oxidized LDL in obese individuals	Curcumin C3 Complex® + BioPerine® (1000 mg + 10 mg/day)
Investigation of the effects of curcumin on serum cytokines in obese individuals: a randomized, controlled trial	Curcumin C3 Complex® + BioPerine® (1000 mg + 10 mg/day)
An investigation of the effects of curcumin on anxiety and depression in obese individuals: a randomized controlled trial	Curcumin C3 Complex® + BioPerine® (1000 mg + 10 mg/day)

Chapter 6
LONG-TERM SAFETY OF PIPERINE

Study Title	Dosage
Lipid-modifying effects of adjunctive therapy with curcuminoids-piperine combination in patients with metabolic syndrome: results of a randomized controlled trial	Curcumin C3 Complex® + BioPerine® (1000 mg + 10 mg/day)
Antioxidant and anti-inflammatory effects of curcuminoids-piperine combination in subjects with metabolic syndrome: a randomized controlled trial and an updated meta-analysis	Curcumin C3 Complex® + BioPerine® (1000 mg + 10 mg/day)
Influence of piperine on the pharmacokinetics of curcumin in animals and human volunteers	Curcumin C3 Complex® + BioPerine® (2000 mg + 20 mg/day)
Effect of a herbal extract containing curcumin and piperine on midazolam, flurbiprofen and paracetamol (acetaminophen) pharmacokinetics in healthy volunteers	Curcumin C3 Complex® + BioPerine® (500 mg + 3 mg) given 4 times over 2 days before drug administration
Effects of supplementation with curcumin on serum adipokine concentrations: a randomized controlled trial	Curcumin C3 Complex® + BioPerine® (1000 mg + 10 mg/day)
Effects of curcumin on serum cytokine concentrations in subjects with metabolic syndrome: a post-hoc analysis of a randomized controlled trial	Curcumin C3 Complex® + BioPerine® (1000 mg + 10 mg/day)
Adjunctive therapy with curcumin for peptic ulcer: a randomized, controlled trial	Curcumin C3 Complex® + BioPerine® (500 mg + 5 mg/day)
Piperine derived from black pepper increases the plasma levels of coenzyme Q10 following oral supplementation	Coenzyme Q10 + BioPerine® (90 or 120 mg + 5 mg/day)
Piperine, an alkaloid derived from black pepper increases serum response of beta-carotene during 14- days of oral beta-carotene supplementation	β–Carotene + BioPerine® (15 mg + 5 mg/day)
Influence of exercise training with resveratrol supplementation on skeletal muscle mitochondrial capacity	Resveratrol + BioPerine® (500 mg + 10 mg/day)
A clinical study on iron deficiency anaemia with BioIron	BioIron tablet (containing 8.5 mg of elemental iron and 2.5 mg of BioPerine®) twice a day
Compositions and methods containing bioavailable Se-Methyl-L-Selenocysteine for human and veterinary use	Se-methyl-L-selenocysteine + BioPerine® (100 µg of elemental selenium + 5 mg piperine/day)
Antioxidant effects of curcuminoids in patients with type 2 diabetes mellitus: a randomized controlled trial	Curcumin C3 Complex® + BioPerine® (1000 mg + 10 mg/day)

Table 23: List of various publications based on several clinical trials using BioPerine®.

Overall, safety of piperine could be supported by following reasons:

- Black pepper, its preparations and piperine have a long history of food use
- No adverse effects have been reported in humans when piperine was consumed in the range of 18.0–32.3 mg/day
- Experimental studies have proved the safety of piperine, which include acute, sub-acute and chronic genotoxicity studies
- Regulatory agencies, including FDA, the Joint FAO/WHO Expert Committee on Food Additives (JECFA) have documented about the use of piperine in various foodstuffs (e.g. baked goods, breakfast cereals, cheese, egg products, soups, snack foods, soft & hard candy, chewing gum, granulated sugar, seasonings and flavor)

Chapter 6 | LONG-TERM SAFETY OF PIPERINE

BioPerine®: Reconciling Traditional Knowledge with Modern Benefits

It has been very well documented that since ancient times, black pepper is an integral part of human diet and is one of the most commonly used spices worldwide. However, today, modern drug discovery process has guided a radical change in the way health benefits of black pepper, and in turn that of piperine, are perceived. Subsequently, piperine is no more just a spice, but is being considered as a food supplement, thermonutrient and as a natural bioenhancer.

BioPerine®, from Sabinsa Corporation, is the only product sourced out of black pepper to obtain a patented status for its ability to increase the bioavailability of nutritional compounds. It has been well recognized as a bioavailability enhancer for nearly two decades, and it is the only source of black pepper to have undergone clinical studies in the United States and several other countries, which substantiate its safety and efficacy for nutritional use.

The doses of BioPerine® recommended for bioavailability enhancement are relatively low when compared to the toxic doses. This translates to a dose of pure piperine in a range of 2.5–15 mg per dose, which equates to an average daily dose of 0.04–0.25* mg of piperine/kg (Table 24).

Recommendation	mg/person*	mg/kg**
BioPerine® daily consumption	2.5–15	0.04–0.25

*Daily dose (1–3 times) was calculated based on the lowest and highest estimated dose of BioPerine® used as a bioenhancing supplement
**Average human weight estimated at 60 kg

Table 24: Estimated daily human consumption of BioPerine®.

BioPerine® and GRAS Status

BioPerine®, a natural bioavailability enhancer from Sabinsa, has received GRAS status after a comprehensive review of safety and toxicology data by an independent panel of scientists with international repute.

Based on the scientific procedures and available comprehensive scientific literature, including human and animal data to determine safety-in-use for black pepper extract (BioPerine®), Expert Panel supported the determination of its GRAS status.

Thus, based on the critical evaluation of the pertinent data and information it was determined that addition of BioPerine®, primarily containing piperine, to the selected foods, such as baked goods, breakfast cereals, milk products, cheese, egg products, processed vegetables, soft candy, soups, snack foods, beverages type I-non-alcoholic, imitation dairy products, hard candy, chewing gum, granulated sugar, seasonings and flavor is GRAS.

GRAS Status: April 2010 (as a flavoring agent)

Safety Level: 13.32 mg/person/per day is **safe**

Sabinsa's Intellectual Property Portfolio on BioPerine®

Prior to Sabinsa's introduction of BioPerine®, utility of black pepper extract as a bioavailability enhancement ingredient in nutritional supplement formulas was scant. The enormous investment in terms of time and resources helped us to determine bioavailability enhancing property of 95% purified piperine, a pungent principle of black pepper (*Piper nigrum*), when administered with wide range of dietary ingredients. These findings in turn helped Sabinsa to obtain seven patents on BioPerine®, with its clearly novel use and process. These patents are strictly enforced in the United States (**US 5,536,506; US 5,744,161; US 5,972,382; US 6,054,585**), Canada (**CA 2247467**), Europe (**EP 0810868**) and Japan (**JP 3953513**).

These patents were issued for compositions and methods for the improvement of gastrointestinal absorption and systemic utilization of nutrients and nutritional supplements by piperine as well as new process for the extraction and purification of piperine. The US Patent office's formal review on BioPerine® in 2006 further reaffirmed that BioPerine® is the only black pepper extract that can legally be used in nutritional supplements for the purpose of enhancing the bioavailability of nutrients and the primary reason for using this in any nutritional formulation.

Trademarks

BioPerine® is also represented by the following trademarks:

United States

Registration Number: 4099964

Representation: BioPerine®

Registration Number: 1976029

Representation: BIOPERINE®

Europe

Registration Number: 000286922

Representation: BIOPERINE®

Japan

Registration Number: 4184700

Representation: BIOPERINE®

Analytical Profile

i. Identification

CAS Registry Number:
94-62-2

IUPAC Name:
(2E,4E)-5-(1,3-Benzodioxol-5-yl)-1-(1-piperidinyl)-2,4-pentadien-1-one

Other Names:
(E,E)-5-(3,4-Methylenedioxyphenyl)-2,4-pentadienoylpiperidide; 1-Piperoylpiperidine; BioPerine®; NSC 21727; Piperin; Piperine

Molecular Formula:
$C_{17}H_{19}NO_3$

Molecular Weight:
285.34

Molecular Structure:

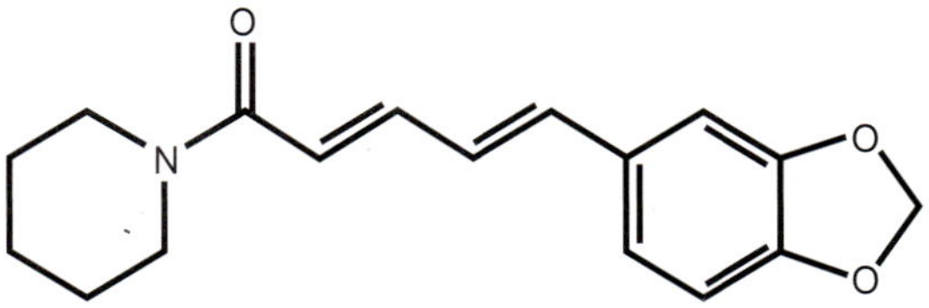

Appearance:
Pale yellow crystalline powder

ANALYTICAL PROFILE

Melting Point:
128–131 °C

Solubility:
Soluble in chloroform, dichloromethane, methanol, ethyl acetate, ethanol, acetone and acetic acid; insoluble in water.

Taste:
Tasteless at first, but induces pungent sensation after a few seconds.

pK_a (18 °C):
12.22

Crystal Nature:
Piperine forms monoclinic prisms from ethanol.

ii. Spectral Data

Ultraviolet (UV) Spectrum
The UV spectrum of BioPerine® in acetonitrile in the region of 200–600 nm exhibits absorption maximum at about 340 nm (ε=32000). The UV spectrum is given in Appendix I.

Infrared (IR) Spectrum
Infrared spectrum of BioPerine® was recorded on a PerkinElmer FT-IR spectrometer by Horizontal Attenuated Total Reflectance (HATR) sampling technique using Zinc Selenide crystal. The IR spectrum is given in Appendix II.

The IR band assignments are given below:
IR (HATR) 2941, 1632, 1581, 1490, 1431, 1250
1192, 1132, 995, 927, 846, 830, 803, 606 cm^{-1}

Wave Number (cm⁻¹)	Assignments
2941	C-H stretching
1632	C=O stretching of conjugated *tert* amide
1581, 1490	C=C (Aromatic) stretch
1250, 1192	=C-O-C asymmetrical stretch
995 / 927	*trans* double bond C-H out of plane bending
846	Out of plane C-H bending of isolated hydrogen of 1,2,4-trisubstituted phenyl
830, 803	Out of plane C-H bending of adjacent hydrogens of 1,2,4-trisubstituted phenyl

¹H Nuclear Magnetic Resonance Spectrum

The ¹H nuclear magnetic resonance (NMR) spectrum of BioPerine® in $CDCl_3$ containing tetramethylsilane (TMS) as internal standard was recorded on a Varian 300 MHz FT-NMR spectrometer. The spectrum is given in Appendix III. The proton signal assignments are given below:

δ (ppm)	Multiplicity	Number of H	Assignment
1.54 – 1.66	m	6	$C_{3''}$-H₂, $C_{4''}$-H₂ & $C_{5''}$-H₂
3.53 – 3.61	br d	4	$C_{2''}$-H₂ & $C_{6''}$-H₂
5.96	s	2	-O-CH₂-O-
6.44	d (J=14.4 Hz)	1	C_2-H
6.72 – 6.77	m	3	C_4-H, C_5-H & $C_{5'}$-H
6.88	dd (J=8.0 Hz, 1.5 Hz)	1	$C_{6'}$-H
6.97	d (J=1.5 Hz)	1	$C_{2'}$-H
7.36 – 7.44	m	1	C_3-H

^{13}C Nuclear Magnetic Resonance Spectrum

The ^{13}C NMR spectrum of BioPerine® in CDCl$_3$ containing TMS as internal standard was recorded on a Varian 75 MHz FT-NMR spectrometer. The spectrum is given in Appendix IV. The carbon signal assignments are given below:

δ (ppm)	Assignment	δ (ppm)	Assignment
24.71	$C_{4''}$	122.55	C_4
25.69	$C_{3''}$	125.40	$C_{6'}$
26.78	$C_{5''}$	131.03	$C_{1'}$
43.27	$C_{2''}$	138.23	C_5
46.93	$C_{6''}$	142.50	C_3
101.34	-O-$\underline{C}$H$_2$-O-	148.16	$C_{3'}$
105.69	$C_{2'}$	148.23	$C_{4'}$
108.51	$C_{5'}$	165.43	C_1
120.13	C_2		

Mass Spectrum

The mass spectrum was recorded on Thermo-Finnigan LCQ Advantage Max (Ion trap) LCMS using Atmospheric Pressure Chemical Ionisation (positive mode); [M+H]$^+$ appears as base peak at m/e 286. The mass spectrum is given in Appendix V.

iii. Elemental Analysis

A typical elemental analysis of a sample of BioPerine® is given below:

Element	Calculated Value (%)	Observed Value (%)
C	71.55	71.40
H	6.71	7.06
N	4.91	4.82

iv. Chromatographic Analysis

High-performance Thin Layer Chromatography

The following high-performance thin layer chromatography (HPTLC) procedure is used for estimation of the purity of BioPerine®. It separates impurities, if any.

- Mobile Phase: Hexane/Acetone (1:1 v/v)

- Stationary Phase: Precoated silica gel plates (GF 254)

- Sample Preparation: Dissolve 25 mg of sample (BioPerine®) in 5 ml of chloroform. Pipette 2 ml sample into a 100 ml volumetric flask and dilute with chloroform to volume

- Standard Preparation: Dissolve 25 mg of piperine (reference standard) in 5 ml chloroform. Pipette 2 ml standard into a 100 ml volumetric flask and dilute with chloroform to volume

- Procedure: Spot separately 20 µl standard preparation, sample preparation and develop the chromatogram to 75% of the plate length. Remove the plate from the developing chamber, mark the solvent front and allow the solvent to evaporate

- Detection: Examine the plate under short wavelength of UV light (254 nm). No spot other than the principal spot in the chromatogram of the solution should be larger or more intense than corresponding spot in the standard solution. Retention factor (R_f) of piperine/BioPerine® is 0.45

High-performance Liquid Chromatography

The following HPLC method is used to estimate the content of BioPerine® in a given sample:

- Mobile Phase: Acetonitrile/Water (50:50); filter and degas

- Standard Preparation: Weigh accurately 50 mg of reference standard of piperine. Transfer into a 100 ml volumetric flask and add 10 ml acetonitrile. Shake and sonicate to dissolve, and dilute to volume with acetonitrile. Pipette out 5 ml of the above solution into a 50 ml volumetric flask and dilute to volume with acetonitrile

- Sample Preparation: Weigh accurately 50 mg of BioPerine® sample. Transfer into a 100 ml volumetric flask and add 10 ml acetonitrile. Shake and sonicate to dissolve, and dilute to volume with acetonitrile. Pipette out 5 ml of above solution into a 50 ml volumetric flask and dilute to volume with acetonitrile

- Procedure: Inject 20 µl of acetonitrile into the HPLC chromatograph as blank. Separately inject 20 µl of standard preparation (3 replicates) and sample preparation in duplicate into the HPLC. Record the response of the major peak due to the analyte in each injection

Calculation:

$$\frac{\text{Area of the sample} \times \text{Standard concentration (mg/ml)} \times \text{Assay of the standard}}{\text{Area of the standard} \times \text{Sample concentration (mg/ml)}}$$

The HPLC profile is given in Appendix VI.

ANALYTICAL PROFILE

APPENDIX - I
UV Spectrum of BioPerine® (Acetonitrile)

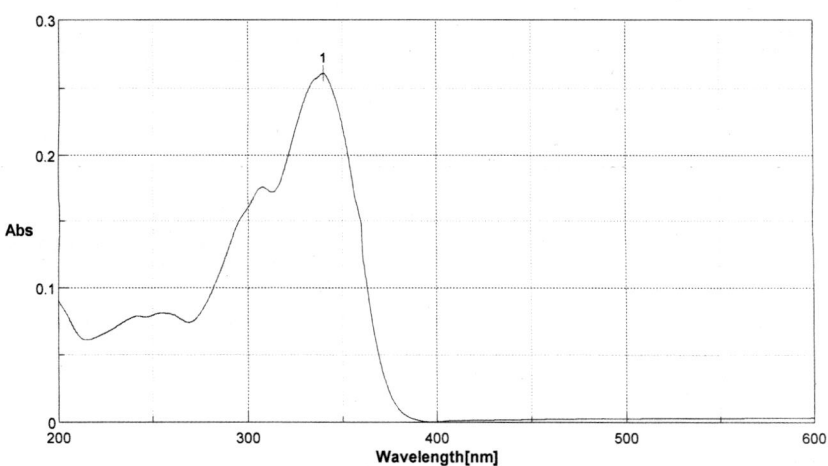

APPENDIX - II
IR Spectrum of BioPerine® (HATR-Zn Se)

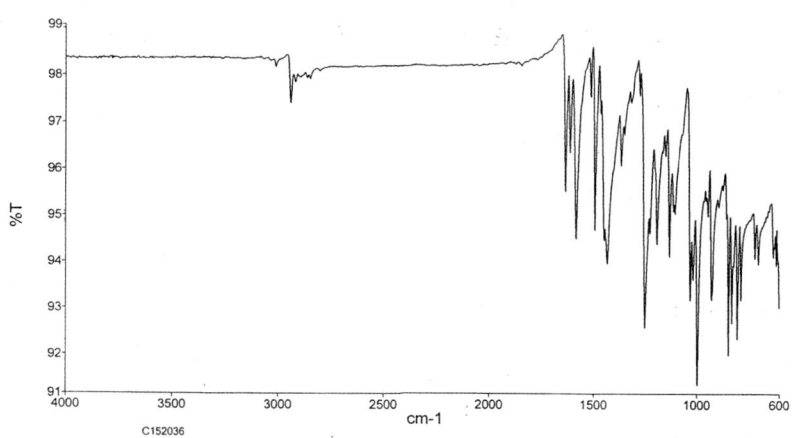

APPENDIX - III
^{1}H NMR Spectrum of BioPerine® (CDCl$_3$, 300 MHz)

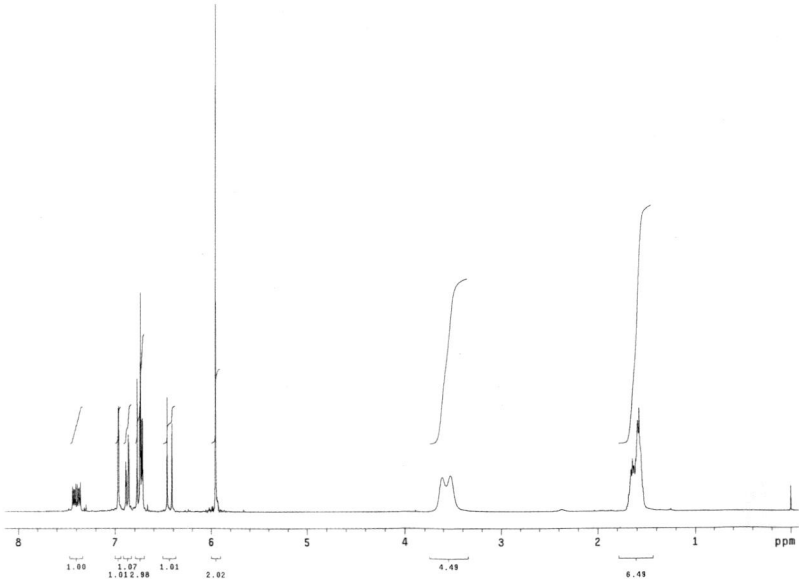

APPENDIX - IV
^{13}C NMR Spectrum of BioPerine® (CDCl$_3$, 75 MHz)

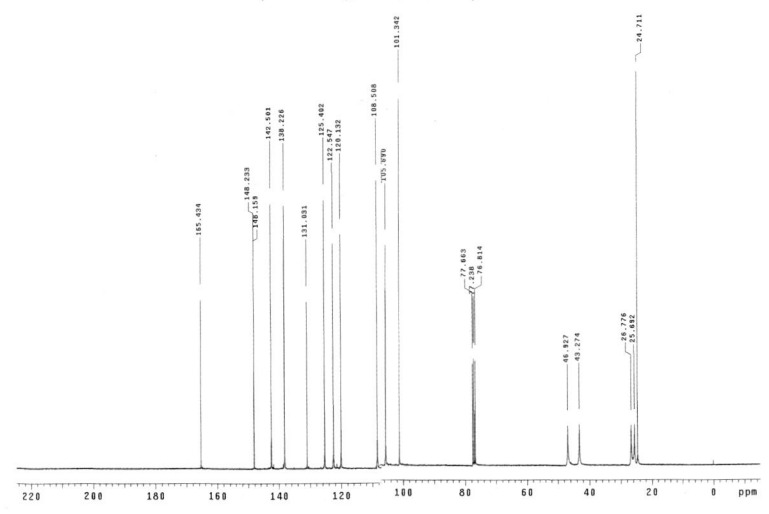

APPENDIX - V
Mass Spectrum of BioPerine® (+APCI)

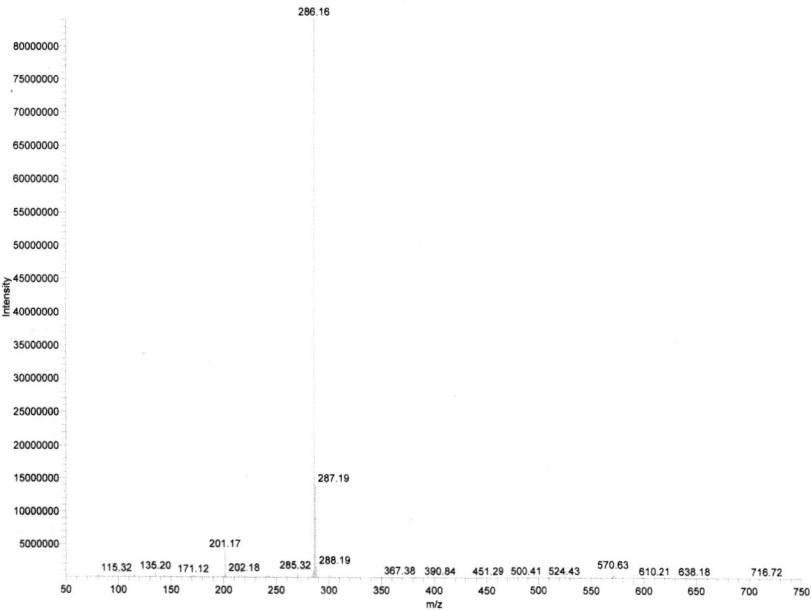

APPENDIX - VI
High-performance Liquid Chromatography of BioPerine®

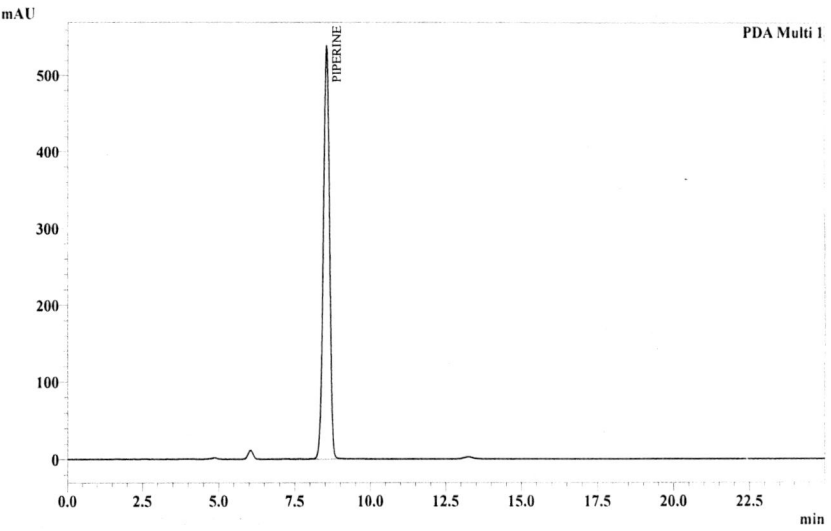

Conclusion

It is certainly apparent that since prehistoric era, human beings have had enormous knowledge about the medicinal potential of natural products, such as plants, herbs and spices. Natural products, being the sole means of treating ailments and injuries, our earliest ancestors, for example, relied upon certain herbs to relieve pain by chewing them or got rid of certain wounds and injuries by wrapping around particular type of leaves.

Natural products have been a significant manifestation of the human evolution, for both medicine as well as health and wellness—precedes recorded human history, probably by thousands of years. Use of plants as medicines may be traced as early as 60,000 years, for example, according to palaeoanthropological studies carried out at the cave site of Shanidar (located in the Zagros Mountains of Kurdistan), Iraq. Neanderthals were believed to have had the wisdom of medicinal properties of several plants (Solecki, 1975).

Hence, it would be reasonable to presume that nearly every civilization of humankind has discovered and made immense use of accumulated experience and knowledge of natural compounds over the ensuing millennia—attributed to their diverse biological activities and varied health benefits.

CONCLUSION

Black pepper is one such spice, which has been an essential part of human diets and commerce. Since time immemorial, black pepper, which holds rich phytochemicals that includes volatile oil, oleoresins and alkaloids, as well as piperine, the main active ingredient with proven clinical effects, is considered as an important healthy food with many pharmacological effects and numerous biological advantages.

Despite its extensive use in the Orient and Occident, the specific identity of the chemicals in black pepper that had the desired therapeutic effects was not known until the 18th and 19th centuries. It was then a widespread recognition of its *diet-health* connection was divulged and its dietary importance was apprecated.

A renewed interest in understanding the health-promoting benefits, diversity in biological activities and drug-like properties of piperine was evident during the past few decades after the advancement in the field of drug discovery and drug development.

As a result, scientific basis of several activities of black pepper and its principal active constituent, piperine, was established pharmacologically (*in vitro, in vivo* and clinical) with well defined experimental protocols as used in modern drug development, which were otherwise not studied in traditional systems of medicine. Several studies have been reported during the last couple of decades, many of which are encouraging and supported some of the clinical uses in traditional systems of medicine, including Ayurveda.

Several systematic pharmacological studies on piperine have revealed its antioxidant, anti-inflammatory, anticancer, anti-obesity, antidiabetic, CNS-related (cognitive enhancement, antidepressant, anxiolytic, anticonvulsant) properties as well as cardiovascular (antihypertensive, antihyperlipidemic) effects and respiratory health support. Piperine has also been found to have beneficial effects on one's digestive system, and very fruitful ergogenic effects, in terms of optimal health and physical performance or overall endurance, not only of hard-core athletes but also people who are ardent to maintain a healthy lifestyle.

Moreover, synergistic interaction with a range of nutrients, minerals, vitamins and other modern therapeutic agents is a renowned and well-established property of piperine.

CONCLUSION

Likewise, characteristic qualities of piperine were scientifically proved to have a broader effect on our bodies than just a pleasant sensory perception. This 'hot' taste of piperine has been attributed to add nutritive value to a variety of phytonutrients and other drugs by enhancing their bioavailability and thermogenesis.

As far as safety of long-term consumption of piperine is concerned, safety data from several animal studies and observations from human exposure have conclusively asserted that the amount of piperine consumed daily in the diet by an average individual is absolutely safe. This can further be ascertained with the fact that FDA has recognized black pepper as GRAS for its intended use as a spice, seasoning and flavoring—which demonstrates safety of long-term use of piperine in daily diet.

As per toxicity studies, dose of piperine, which has been known to increase the bioavailability of the various bioactives, is several times lower than the estimated amount of piperine consumed daily in the diet by an average individual in the United States. Additionally, non-genotoxic nature of piperine, as observed by several researchers, further reinforces its safety profile.

Sabinsa's BioPerine® is one such product standardized to 95% piperine and is the only product sourced out of black pepper to obtain a patented status for its bioenhancing property of nutrients, and is the only source from black pepper to get validated for its safety and efficacy for nutritional use.

Overall, given that black pepper is the most revered spice that has been consumed for millennia, it would appear to be exceptionally safe and displays a vast array of health benefits. Thus, it promises maximum benefit and potency in promoting overall health and well being, improving bioavailability of co-administered agents as well as in preventing and/or use in the therapy of various ailments.

References

Abdelhamed S, Yokoyama S, Refaat A, Ogura K, Yagita H, Awale S et al. Piperine enhances the efficacy of TRAIL-based therapy for triple-negative breast cancer cells. *Anticancer Res*. 2014;34(4):1893–9.

Ahmad N, Fazal H, Abbasi BH, Farooq S, Ali M, Khan MA. Biological role of *Piper nigrum* L. (Black pepper): A Review. *Asian Pac J Trop Biomed*. 2012; S1945–53.

Amin ML. P-glycoprotein inhibition for optimal drug delivery. *Drug Target Insights*. 2013;7:27–34.

Anonymous. Available at: http://www.rediff.com/money/2007/may/29pep.htm. Accessed on: 08 Novmeber 2016.

Aswar U, Shintre S, Chepurwar S, Aswar M. Antiallergic effect of piperine on ovalbumin-induced allergic rhinitis in mice. *Pharm Biol*. 2015;53(9):1358–66.

Atal CK, Zutshi U, Rao PG. Scientific evidence on the role of Ayurvedic herbals on bioavailability of drugs. *J Ethnopharmacol*.1981;4(2):229–32.

Atal CK, Dubey RK, Singh J. Biochemical basis of enhanced drug bioavailability by piperine: evidence that piperine is a potent inhibitor of drug metabolism. *J Pharmacol Exp Ther*. 1985;232(1):258–62.

Atal N, Bedi KL. Bioenhancers: Revolutionary concept to market. *J Ayurveda Integr Med*. 2010;1(2):96–9.

Atal S, Agrawal RP, Vyas S, Phadnis P, Rai N. Evaluation of the effect of piperine per se on blood glucose level in alloxan-induced diabetic mice. *Acta Pol Pharm*. 2012;69(5):965–9.

Atal S, Atal S, Vyas S, Phadnis P. Bioenhancing effect of piperine with metformin on lowering blood glucose level in alloxan induced diabetic mice. *Pharmacognosy Res*. 2016; 8(1):56–60.

Badmaev V, Majeed M, Norkus EP. Piperine, an alkaloid derived from black pepper increases serum response of beta-carotene during 14-days of oral beta-carotene supplementation. *Nutr Res*. 1999;19(3):381–8.

Badmaev V, Majeed M, Prakash L. Piperine derived from black pepper increases the plasma levels of coenzyme Q10 following oral supplementation. *J Nutr Biochem*. 2000;11(2):109–13.

Bae GS, Kim MS, Jung WS, Seo SW, Yun SW, Kim SG et al. Inhibition of lipopolysaccharide-induced inflammatory responses by piperine. *Eur J Pharmacol*. 2010;642 (1–3):154–62.

REFERENCES

Bae GS, Kim MS, Jeong J, Lee HY, Park KC, Koo BS et al. Piperine ameliorates the severity of cerulein-induced acute pancreatitis by inhibiting the activation of mitogen activated protein kinases. *Biochem Biophys Res Commun*. 2011;410(3):382–8.

Bae GS, Kim JJ, Park KC, Koo BS, Jo IJ, Choi SB et al. Piperine inhibits lipopolysaccharide-induced maturation of bone-marrow-derived dendritic cells through inhibition of ERK and JNK activation. *Phytother Res*. 2012;26(12):1893–7.

Bajad S, Bedi KL, Singla AK, Johri RK. Piperine inhibits gastric emptying and gastrointestinal transit in rats and mice. *Planta Med*. 2001;67(2):176–9.

Bajad S, Coumar M, Khajuria R, Suri OP, Bedi KL. Characterization of a new rat urinary metabolite of piperine by LC/NMR/MS studies. *Eur J Pharm Sci*. 2003;19(5):413–21.

Bang JS, Oh DH, Choi HM, Sur BJ, Lim SJ, Kim JY et al. Anti-inflammatory and antiarthritic effects of piperine in human interleukin 1beta-stimulated fibroblast-like synoviocytes and in rat arthritis models. *Arthritis Res Ther*. 2009. DOI: 10.1186/ar2662.

Banji D, Banji OJ, Dasaroju S, Kranthi KC. Curcumin and piperine abrogate lipid and protein oxidation induced by D-galactose in rat brain. *Brain Res*. 2013a;1515:1–11.

Banji D, Banji OJ, Dasaroju S, Annamalai AR. Piperine and curcumin exhibit synergism in attenuating D-galactose induced senescence in rats. *Eur J Pharmacol*. 2013b;703(1–3):91–9.

Bao XM, Na SS, Lu JK. Studies of effective part group of piperine to regulating lipid [Article in Chinese]. *Zhongguo Zhong Yao Za Zhi*. 2013;38(6):909–13.

Bhardwaj RK, Glaeser H, Becquemont L, Klotz U, Gupta SK, Fromm MF. Piperine, a major constituent of black pepper, inhibits human P-glycoprotein and CYP3A4. *J Pharmacol Exp Ther*. 2002;302(2):645–50.

Bhat BG, Chandrasekhara N. Studies on the metabolism of piperine: absorption, tissue distribution and excretion of urinary conjugates in rats. *Toxicology*. 1986a;40(1):83–92.

Bhat BG, Chandrasekhara N. Lack of adverse influence of black pepper, its oleoresin and piperine in the weanling rat. *J Food Safety*. 1986b;7(4):215–23.

Bhat BG, Chandrasekhara N. Effect of black pepper and piperine on bile secretion and composition in rats. *Nahrung*. 1987a;31(9):913–6.

Bhat BG, Chandrasekhara N. Metabolic disposition of piperine in the rat. *Toxicology*. 1987b;44(1):99–106.

Bhutani MK, Bishnoi M, Kulkarni SK. Anti-depressant like effect of curcumin and its combination with piperine in unpredictable chronic stress-induced behavioral, biochemical and neurochemical changes. *Pharmacol Biochem Behav*. 2009;92(1):39–43.

Bordner J, Mullins P. Piperine, $C_{17}H_{19}NO_3$. *Crystal Structure Comm*. 1974;3(4):693–5.

REFERENCES

BrahmaNaidu P, Nemani H, Meriga B, Mehar SK, Potana S, Ramgopalrao S. Mitigating efficacy of piperine in the physiological derangements of high-fat diet-induced obesity in Sprague Dawley rats. *Chem Biol Interact.* 2014;221:42–51.

Brewer MS. Natural antioxidants: sources, compounds, mechanisms of action, and potential applications. *Compr Rev Food Sci Food Saf.* 2011;10:221–47.

Bukhari IA, Pivac N, Alhumayyd MS, Mahesar AL, Gilani AH. The analgesic and anticonvulsant effects of piperine in mice. *J Physiol Pharmacol.* 2013;64(6):789–94.

Butler S. Off the Spice Rack: The Story of Pepper (2013). Available at: http://www.history.com/news/hungry-history/off-the-spice-rack-the-story-of-pepper. Accessed on: 16 November 2016.

Butt MS, Naz A, Sultan MT, Qayyum MM. Anti-oncogenic perspectives of spices/herbs: A comprehensive review. *EXCLI J.* 2013;12:1043–65.

Capasso R, Izzo AA, Borrelli F, Russo A, Sautebin L, Pinto A et al. Effect of piperine, the active ingredient of black pepper, on intestinal secretion in mice. *Life Sci.* 2002;71(19):2311–7.

Chen CY, Li W, Qu KP, Chen CR. Piperine exerts antiseizure effects via the TRPV1 receptor in mice. *Eur J Pharmacol.* 2013;714(1–3):288–94.

Chen YF, Wang YW, Huang WS, Lee MM, Wood WG, Leung YM et al. *Trans*-cinnamaldehyde, an essential oil in cinnamon powder, ameliorates cerebral ischemia-induced brain injury via inhibition of neuroinflammation through attenuation of iNOS, COX-2 expression and NF-κB signaling pathway. *Neuromolecular Med.* 2016;18(3):322–33.

Chonpathompikunlert P, Wattanathorn J, Muchimapura S. Piperine, the main alkaloid of Thai black pepper, protects against neurodegeneration and cognitive impairment in animal model of cognitive deficit like condition of Alzheimer's disease. *Food Chem Toxicol.* 2010;48(3):798–802.

Claus H, Gerhard S. Piperine—an example of individually different (polymorph) metabolism of an omnipresent nutrition component. *Liebigs Ann Chem.* 1984;1319–31.

Code of Federal Regulations. Title 21-Food and Drugs, Substances Generally Recognized As Safe (2016). Available at: http://www.accessdata.fda.gov/scripts/cdrh/cfdocs/cfcfr/CFRSearch.cfm?fr=182.20. Accessed on: 23 September 2013.

Concon JM, Newburg DS, Swerczek T. Black pepper (*Piper nigrum*): Evidence of carcinogenicity. *Nutr Cancer.* 1979;1(3):22–6.

da Cruz GM, Felipe CF, Scorza FA, da Costa MA, Tavares AF, Menezes ML et al. Piperine decreases pilocarpine-induced convulsions by GABAergic mechanisms. *Pharmacol Biochem Behav.* 2013;104:144–53.

Daware MB, Mujumdar AM, Ghaskadbi S. Reproductive toxicity of piperine in Swiss albino mice. *Planta Med.* 2000;66(3):231–6.

REFERENCES

Delecroix B, Abaïdia AE, Leduc C, Dawson B, Dupont G. Curcumin and piperine supplementation and recovery following exercise induced muscle damage: A randomized controlled trial. *J Sports Sci Med*. 2017;16(1):147–53.

de Souza Grinevicius VM, Kviecinski MR, Santos Mota NS, Ourique F, Porfirio Will Castro LS, Andreguetti RR *et al*. *Piper nigrum* ethanolic extract rich in piperamides causes ROS overproduction, oxidative damage in DNA leading to cell cycle arrest and apoptosis in cancer cells. *J Ethnopharmacol*. 2016;189:139–47.

Deepak V, Kruger MC, Joubert A, Coetzee M. Piperine alleviates osteoclast formation through the p38/c-Fos/NFATc1 signaling axis. *Biofactors*. 2015;41(6):403–13.

D'Hooge R, Pei YQ, Raes A, Lebrun P, van Bogaert PP, de Deyn PP. Anticonvulsant activity of piperine on seizures induced by excitatory amino acid receptor agonists. *Arzneimittelforschung*. 1996;46(6):557–60.

Di X, Wang X, Di X, Liu Y. Effect of piperine on the bioavailability and pharmacokinetics of emodin in rats. *J Pharm Biomed Anal*. 2015;115:144–9.

Diwan V, Poudyal H, Brown L. Piperine attenuates cardiovascular, liver and metabolic changes in high carbohydrate, high-fat-fed rats. *Cell Biochem Biophys*. 2013;67(2):297–304.

Do MT, Kim HG, Choi JH, Khanal T, Park BH, Tran TP *et al*. Antitumor efficacy of piperine in the treatment of human HER2-overexpressing breast cancer cells. *Food Chem*. 2013;141(3):2591–9.

Dogra RK, Khanna S, Shanker R. Immunotoxicological effects of piperine in mice. *Toxicology*. 2004;196(3):229–36.

Dong Y, Huihui Z, Li C. Piperine inhibit inflammation, alveolar bone loss and collagen fibers breakdown in a rat periodontitis model. *J Periodontal Res*. 2015;50(6):758–65.

Doucette CD, Hilchie AL, Liwski R, Hoskin DW. Piperine, a dietary phytochemical, inhibits angiogenesis. *J Nutr Biochem*. 2013;24(1):231–9.

Doucette CD, Rodgers G, Liwski RS, Hoskin DW. Piperine from black pepper inhibits activation-induced proliferation and effector function of T lymphocytes. *J Cell Biochem*. 2015;116(11):2577–88.

Duangjai A, Ingkaninan K, Praputbut S, Limpeanchob N. Black pepper and piperine reduce cholesterol uptake and enhance translocation of cholesterol transporter proteins. *J Nat Med*. 2013;67(2):303–10.

Dudhatra GB, Mody SK, Awale MM, Patel HB, Modi CM, Kumar A *et al*. A comprehensive review on pharmacotherapeutics of herbal bioenhancers. *Scientific World J*. 2012. DOI: 10.1100/2012/637953.

Dutta M, Ghosh AK, Mishra P, Jain G, Rangari V, Chattopadhyay A *et al*. Protective effects of piperine against copper-ascorbate-induced toxic injury to goat cardiac mitochondria *in vitro*. *Food Funct*. 2014;5(9):2252–67.

Esmaily H, Sahebkar A, Iranshahi M, Ganjali S, Mohammadi A, Ferns G *et al*. An investigation of the effects of curcumin on anxiety and depression in obese individuals: a randomized controlled trial. *Chin J Integr Med*. 2015;21(5):332–8.

REFERENCES

Feng X, Liu Y, Wang X, Di X. Effects of piperine on the intestinal permeability and pharmacokinetics of linarin in rats. *Molecules*. 2014;19(5):5624–33.

Fernández S, Wasowski C, Paladini AC, Marder M. Sedative and sleep-enhancing properties of linarin, a flavonoid-isolated from *Valeriana officinalis*. *Pharmacol Biochem Behav*. 2004;77(2):399–404.

Fofaria NM, Kim SH, Srivastava SK. Piperine causes G1 phase cell cycle arrest and apoptosis in melanoma cells through checkpoint kinase-1 activation. *PLoS One*. 2014. DOI: 10.1371/journal.pone.0094298.

Fu M, Sun ZH, Zuo HC. Neuroprotective effect of piperine on primarily cultured hippocampal neurons. *Biol Pharm Bull*. 2010;33(4):598–603.

Geppetti P, Trevisani M. Activation of sensitization of the vanilloid receptor: role in gastrointestinal inflammation and function. *Br J Pharmacol*. 2004;141(8):1313–20.

Gilhotra N, Dhingra D. Possible involvement of GABAergic and nitriergic systems for antianxiety-like activity of piperine in unstressed and stressed mice. *Pharmacol Rep*. 2014;66(5):885–91.

Glatzel H. Physiological aspects of flavour compounds. *Bibl Nutr Dieta*. 1967;9:71–86.

Gordo SM, Pinheiro DG, Moreira EC, Rodrigues SM, Poltronieri MC, de Lemos OF *et al*. High-throughput sequencing of black pepper root transcriptome. *BMC Plant Biol*. 2012. DOI: 10.1186/1471-2229-12-168.

Greenshields AL, Doucette CD, Sutton KM, Madera L, Annan H, Yaffe PB *et al*. Piperine inhibits the growth and motility of triplenegative breast cancer cells. *Cancer Lett*. 2015;357(1):129–40.

Gülçin I. The antioxidant and radical scavenging activities of black pepper (*Piper nigrum*) seeds. *Int J Food Sci Nutr*. 2005;56(7):491–9.

Gupta RA, Motiwala MN, Dumore NG, Danao KR, Ganjare AB. Effect of piperine on inhibition of FFA-induced TLR4-mediated inflammation and amelioration of acetic acid-induced ulcerative colitis in mice. *J Ethnopharmacol*. 2015;164:239–46.

Han HK. The effects of black pepper on the intestinal absorption and hepatic metabolism of drugs. *Expert Opin Drug Metab Toxicol*. 2011;7(6):721–9.

Han Y, Chin Tan TM, Lim LY. *In vitro* and *in vivo* evaluation of the effects of piperine on P-gp function and expression. *Toxicol Appl Pharmacol*. 2008;230(3):283–9.

Harrison J. History of Spices in India (2016). Available at: http://thespicejournal.com/spice-producing-countries/india/history-of-spices-in-india/. Accessed on: 16 November 2016.

Hee KY, Boo CK, Seok KT, Hyun YI, Woo NS, inventors; Pulmuone Holdings Co. Ltd., assignee. Compound containing piperine for promoting absorption of *Panax ginseng* saponin. *Republic of Korean Patent* KR101281827B1. 2013 July 03.

REFERENCES

Hiwale AR, Dhuley JN, Naik SR. Effect of co-administration of piperine on pharmacokinetics of beta-lactam antibiotics in rats. *Indian J Exp Biol*. 2002;40(3):277–81.

Hlavačková L, Urbanova A, Uličná O, Janega P, Cerná A, Babál P. Piperine, active substance of black pepper, alleviates hypertension induced by NO synthase inhibition. *Bratisl Lek Listy*. 2010;111(8):426–31.

Hlavačková L, Janegová A, Uličná O, Janega P, Cerná A, Babál P. Spice up the hypertension diet – curcumin and piperine prevent remodeling of aorta in experimental L-NAME induced hypertension. *Nutr Metab*. 2011. DOI: 10.1186/1743-7075-8-72.

Hollander JM, Mechanick JI. Complementary and alternative medicine and the management of the metabolic syndrome. *J Am Diet Assoc*. 2008;108(3):495–509.

Holzer P. TRP channels in the digestive system. *Curr Pharm Biotechnol*. 2011a;12(1):24–34.

Holzer P. Transient receptor potential (TRP) channels as drug targets for diseases of the digestive system. *Pharmacol Ther*. 2011b;131(1):142–70.

Hou XF, Pan H, Xu LH, Zha QB, He XH, Ouyang DY. Piperine suppresses the expression of CXCL8 in lipopolysaccharide-activated SW480 and HT29 cells via downregulating the mitogen-activated protein kinase pathways. *Inflammation*. 2015;38(3):1093–102.

Hu D, Wang Y, Chen Z, Ma Z, You Q, Zhang X et al. The protective effect of piperine on dextran sulfate sodium-induced inflammatory bowel disease and its relation with pregnane X receptor activation. *J Ethnopharmacol*. 2015;169:109–23.

Hu Y, Liao HB, Liu P, Guo DH, Wang YY. Antidepressant effects of piperine and its neuroprotective mechanism in rats [Article in Chinese]. *Zhong Xi Yi Jie He Xue Bao*. 2009;7(7):667–70.

Huang W, Chen Z, Wang Q, Lin M, Wu S, Yan Q et al. Piperine potentiates the antidepressant-like effect of *trans*-resveratrol: involvement of monoaminergic system. *Metab Brain Dis*. 2013;28(4):585–95.

Izzo AA, Capasso R, Pinto L, Di Carlo G, Mascolo N, Capasso F. Effect of vanilloid drugs on gastrointestinal transit in mice. *Br J Pharmacol*. 2001;132(7):1411–6.

Jadhav SA, Prabhavalkar K. Anti-inflammatory activity of *trans*-cinnamaldehyde and piperine combination against carrageenan induced paw edema. *IJPSR*. 2015;6(12):5188–92.

Jadhav SA, Prabhavalkar K. Combination of *trans*-cinnamaldehyde and piperine against complete freund's adjuvant induced arthritis animal model illustrating anti-arthritic activity. *EJBPS*. 2016;3(4):347–54.

Jaffee S. International Spice Market Context. In: Delivering and Taking the Heat: Indian Spices and Evolving Product and Process Standards. (2005). Available at: http://siteresources.worldbank.org/INTRANETTRADE/Resources/Topics/Standards/IndiaSpices.pdf. Accessed on: 17 November 2016.

REFERENCES

Jancova P, Anzenbacher P, Anzenbacherova E. Phase II drug metabolizing enzymes. *Biomed Pap Med Fac Univ Palacky Olomouc Czech Repub.* 2010;154(2):103–16.

Jangra A, Kwatra M, Singh T, Pant R, Kushwah P, Sharma Y et al. Piperine augments the protective effect of curcumin against lipopolysaccharide-induced neurobehavioral and neurochemical deficits in mice. *Inflammation.* 2016;39(3):1025–38.

Jensen-Jarolim E, Gajdzik L, Haberl I, Kraft D, Scheiner O, Graf J. Hot spices influence permeability of human intestinal epithelial monolayers. *J Nutr.* 1998;128(3):577–81.

Jin X, Zhang ZH, Sun E, Tan XB, Li SL, Cheng XD et al. Enhanced oral absorption of 20(S)-protopanaxadiol by self-assembled liquid crystalline nanoparticles containing piperine: *in vitro* and *in vivo* studies. *Int J Nanomedicine.* 2013;8:641–52.

Johnson JJ, Nihal M, Siddiqui IA, Scarlett CO, Bailey HH, Mukhtar H et al. Enhancing the bioavailability of resveratrol by combining it with piperine. *Mol Nutr Food Res.* 2011;55(8):1169–76.

Johri RK, Zutshi U. An Ayurvedic formulation 'Trikatu' and its constituents. *J Ethnopharmacol.* 1992;37(2):85–91.

Johri RK, Thusu N, Khajuria A, Zutshi U. Piperine-mediated changes in the permeability of rat intestinal epithelial cells. The status of gamma-glutamyl transpeptidase activity, uptake of amino acids and lipid peroxidation. *Biochem Pharmacol.* 1992;43(7):1401–7.

Joy N, Abraham Z, Soniya EV. A preliminary assessment of genetic relationships among agronomically important cultivars of black pepper. *BMC Genet.* 2007. DOI:10.1186/1471-2156-8-42.

Jwa H, Choi Y, Park UH, Um SJ, Yoon SK, Park T. Piperine, an LXRα antagonist, protects against hepatic steatosis and improves insulin signaling in mice fed a high-fat diet. *Biochem Pharmacol.* 2012;84(11):1501–10.

Kakalij RM, Kumar BD, Diwan PV. Comparative evaluation of nephroprotective potential of resveratrol and piperine on nephrotic BALB/c mice. *Indian J Pharmacol.* 2016;48(4):382–7.

Kang MJ, Cho JY, Shim BH, Kim DK, Lee J. Bioavailability enhancing activities of natural compounds from medicinal plants. *J Med Plants Res.* 2009;3(13):1204–11.

Kapoor IP, Singh B, Singh G, De Heluani CS, De Lampasona MP, Catalan CA. Chemistry and *in vitro* antioxidant activity of volatile oil and oleoresins of black pepper (*Piper nigrum*). *J Agric Food Chem.* 2009;57(12):5358–64.

Karekar VR, Mujumdar AM, Joshi SS, Dhuley J, Shinde SL, Ghaskadbi S. Assessment of genotoxic effect of piperine using *Salmonella typhimurium* and somatic and somatic and germ cells of Swiss albino mice. *Arzneimittelforschung.* 1996;46(10):972–5.

Kaur G, Meena C. Amelioration of obesity, glucose intolerance, and oxidative stress in high-fat diet and low-dose streptozotocin-induced diabetic rats by combination consisting of "curcumin with piperine and quercetin". *ISRN Pharmacol.* 2012. DOI: 10.5402/2012/957283.

REFERENCES

Kaur G, Invally M, Chintamaneni M. Influence of piperine and quercetin on antidiabetic potential of curcumin. *J Complement Integr Med*. 2016;13(3):247–55.

Kesarwani K, Gupta R, Mukerjee A. Bioavailability enhancers of herbal origin: an overview. *Asian Pac J Trop Biomed*. 2013;3(4):253–66.

Khajuria A, Thusu N, Zutshi U. Piperine modulates permeability characteristics of intestine by inducing alterations in membrane dynamics: influence on brush border membrane fluidity, ultrastructure and enzyme kinetics. *Phytomedicine*. 2002;9(3):224–31.

Khajuria A, Thusu N, Zutshi U, Bedi KL. Piperine modulation of carcinogen induced oxidative stress in intestinal mucosa. *Mol Cell Biochem*. 1998a;189(1–2):113–8.

Khajuria A, Zutshi U, Bedi KL. Permeability characteristics of piperine on oral absorption--an active alkaloid from peppers and a bioavailability enhancer. *Indian J Exp Biol*. 1998b;36(1):46–50.

Khom S, Strommer B, Schöffmann A, Hintersteiner J, Baburin I, Erker T et al. GABAA receptor modulation by piperine and a non-TRPV1 activating derivative. *Biochem Pharmacol*. 2013;85(12):1827–36.

Khonche A, Biglarian O, Panahi Y, Valizadegan G, Soflaei SS, Ghamarchehreh ME et al. Adjunctive therapy with curcumin for peptic ulcer: a randomized controlled trial. *Drug Res* (Stuttg). 2016;66(8):444–8.

Kim DH. Chemical diversity of *Panax ginseng, Panax quinquifolium,* and *Panax notoginseng*. *J Ginseng Res*. 2012;36(1):1–15.

Kim HG, Han EH, Jang WS, Choi JH, Khanal T, Park BH et al. Piperine inhibits PMA-induced cyclooxygenase-2 expression through downregulating NFκB, C/EBP and AP1 signaling pathways in murine macrophages. *Food Chem Toxicol*. 2012;50(7):2342–8.

Kim J. Neuroprotective effect of compound K isolated from fermented Korean Ginseng through stimulation of Nrf2 signaling pathway. *Med Aromat Plants*. 2015. DOI: 10.4172/2167-0412.C1.003.

Kindell SS. Studies on selected genotoxic and toxic properties of piperine. 1984. PhD thesis, Drexel University, Philadelphia, PA.

Koul IB, Kapil A. Evaluation of the liver protective potential of piperine, an active principle of black and long peppers. *Planta Med*. 1993;59(5):413–7.

Krishnakumar N, Manoharan S, Palaniappan PR, Venkatachalam P, Manohar MG. Chemopreventive efficacy of piperine in 7,12-dimethyl benz [a] anthracene (DMBA)-induced hamster buccal pouch carcinogenesis: an FTIR study. *Food Chem Toxicol*. 2009;47(11):2813–20.

Kundu P, Das M, Tripathy K, Sahoo SK. Delivery of dual drug loaded lipid based nanoparticles across the blood-brain barrier impart enhanced neuroprotection in a rotenone induced mouse model of Parkinson's disease. *ACS Chem Neurosci*. 2016. DOI: 10.1021/acschemneuro.6b00207.

REFERENCES

Lai LH, Fu QH, Liu Y, Jiang K, Guo QM, Chen QY et al. Piperine suppresses tumor growth and metastasis in vitro and in vivo in a 4T1 murine breast cancer model. *Acta Pharmacol Sin.* 2012;33(4):523–30.

Lambert JD, Hong J, Kim DH, Mishin VM, Yang CS. Piperine enhances the bioavailability of the tea polyphenol (-)-epigallocatechin-3-gallate in mice. *J Nutr.* 2004;134(8):1948–52.

Li S, Wang C, Wang M, Li W, Matsumoto K, Tang Y. Antidepressant-like effects of piperine in chronic mild stress-treated mice and its possible mechanisms. *Life Sci.* 2007;80(15):1373–81.

Li S, Lei Y, Jia Y, Li N, Wink M, Ma Y. Piperine, a piperidine alkaloid from *Piper nigrum* re-sensitizes P-gp, MRP1 and BCRP dependent multidrug resistant cancer cells. *Phytomedicine.* 2011;19(1):83–7.

Li Y, Li M, Wu S, Tian Y. Combination of curcumin and piperine prevents formation of gallstones in C57BL6 mice fed on lithogenic diet: whether NPC1L1/SREBP2 participates in this process? *Lipids Health Dis.* 2015a. DOI: 10.1186/s12944-015-0106-2.

Li Y, Li K, Hu Y, Xu B, Zhao J. Piperine mediates LPS-induced inflammatory and catabolic effects in rat intervertebral disc. *Int J Clin Exp Pathol.* 2015b;8(6):6203–13.

Lin Y, Xu J, Liao H, Li L, Pan L. Piperine induces apoptosis of lung cancer A549 cells via p53-dependent mitochondrial signaling pathway. *Tumour Biol.* 2014;35(4):3305–10.

Liu Y, Yadev VR, Aggarwal BB, Nair MG. Inhibitory effects of black pepper (*Piper nigrum*) extracts and compounds on human tumor cell proliferation, cyclooxygenase enzymes, lipid peroxidation and nuclear transcription factor-kappaB. *Nat Prod Commun.* 2010;5(8):1253–7.

Liu Y, Zhang Y, Lin K, Zhang DX, Tian M, Guo HY et al. Protective effect of piperine on electrophysiology abnormalities of left atrial myocytes induced by hydrogen peroxide in rabbits. *Life Sci.* 2014;94(2):99–105.

Lu J, Chen Z, Wang Y, Xiao Y, Li W. The mutagenicity of piperine. *Carcinog Teratog Mutagen.* 2009;21(3):241–2.

Lu Y, Liu J, Li H, Gu L. Piperine ameliorates lipopolysaccharide-induced acute lung injury via modulating NF-κB signaling pathways. *Inflammation.* 2016;39(1):303–8.

Lund KC, Pantuso T. Combination effects of quercetin, resveratrol and curcumin on *in vitro* intestinal absorption. *J Restorative Med.* 2014;3(1):112–20.

Ma Y, Tian M, Liu P, Wang Z, Guan Y, Liu Y et al. Piperine effectively protects primary cultured atrial myocytes from oxidative damage in the infant rabbit model. *Mol Med Rep.* 2014;10(5):2627–32.

Madrigal-Bujaidar E, Diaz Barriga S, Mota P, Guzman R, Cassani M. Sister chromatid exchanges induced *in vitro* and *in vivo* by an extract of black pepper. *Food Chem Toxicol.* 1997;35(6):567–71.

Majeed M, Ananthanarayanan N, Nagabhushanam K, Rajendran R, George S, Prakash S, inventors; Sami Labs Ltd., assignee. Compositions and methods containing bioavailable Se-methyl-L-selenocysteine for human and veterinary use. United States Patent US 6,982,273 B1. 2006 January 03.

REFERENCES

Majeed M, Badmaev V, Prakash L. BioPerine®—Nature's own thermonutrient® and Natural bioavailability enhancer. New Jersey: NutriScience Publishers, Inc.; 1999. p. 7–64.

Majeed M, Majeed A (Eds). Curry Powder to Clinical Significance. New Jersey: NutriScience Publishers, LLC; 2015. p. 69–173.

Majeed M, Vaidyanathan P, Kiradi P, Majeed S, Vuppala KK. An evaluation of bioavailability enhancement of organic elemental iron with BioPerine® in rabbits. *Int J Pharm Pharm Res*. 2016a;5(4):72–9.

Majeed M, Vaidyanathan P, Kiradi P, Lad PS, Vuppala KK. A clinical study on iron deficiency anaemia with BioIron. *Int J Ayur Pharma Res*. 2016b;4(10):18–24.

Makhov P, Golovine K, Canter D, Kutikov A, Simhan J, Corlew MM *et al*. Co-administration of piperine and docetaxel results in improved anti-tumor efficacy via inhibition of CYP3A4 activity. *Prostate*. 2012;72(6):661–7.

Mao QQ, Xian YF, Ip SP, Che CT. Involvement of serotonergic system in the antidepressant-like effect of piperine. *Prog Neuropsychopharmacol Biol Psychiatry*. 2011a;35(4):1144–7.

Mao QQ, Huang Z, Ip SP, Xian YF, Che CT. Role of 5HT(1A) and 5HT(1B) receptors in the antidepressant-like effect of piperine in the forced swim test. *Neurosci Lett*. 2011b;504(2):181–4.

Mao QQ, Huang Z, Ip SP, Xian YF, Che CT. Protective effects of piperine against corticosterone-induced neurotoxicity in PC12 cells. *Cell Mol Neurobiol*. 2012;32(4):531–7.

Mao QQ, Huang Z, Zhong XM, Xian YF, Ip SP. Piperine reverses chronic unpredictable mild stress-induced behavioral and biochemical alterations in rats. *Cell Mol Neurobiol*. 2014a;34(3):403–8.

Mao QQ, Huang Z, Zhong XM, Xian YF, Ip SP. Brain-derived neurotrophic factor signalling mediates the antidepressant-like effect of piperine in chronically stressed mice. *Behav Brain Res*. 2014b;261:140–5.

Mao QQ, Huang Z, Zhong XM, Xian YF, Ip SP. Piperine reverses the effects of corticosterone on behavior and hippocampal BDNF expression in mice. *Neurochem Int*. 2014c;74:36–41.

Martins CA, Leyhausen G, Volk J, Geurtsen W. Curcumin in combination with piperine suppresses osteoclastogenesis *in vitro*. *J Endod*. 2015;41(10):1638–45.

McNamara FN, Randall A, Gunthorpe MJ. Effects of piperine, the pungent component of black peppers, at the human vanilloid receptor (TRPV1). *Br J Pharmacol*. 2005;144(6):781–90.

Melissa. A Brief History of Pepper (2014). Available at: http://www.todayifoundout.com/index.php/2014/01/brief-history-pepper/. Accessed on: 16 November 2016.

Micevych PE, Yaksh TL, Szolcsanyi J. Effect of intrathecal capsaicin analogues on the immunofluorescence of peptides and serotonin in the dorsal horn in rats. *Neuroscience*. 1983;8(1):123–31.

REFERENCES

Mishra A, Punia JK, Bladen C, Zamponi GW, Goel RK. Anticonvulsant mechanisms of piperine, a piperidine alkaloid. *Channels* (Austin). 2015;9(5):317–23.

Mittal R, Gupta RL. *In vitro* antioxidant activity of piperine. *Methods Find Exp Clin Pharmacol*. 2000;22(5):271–4.

Mohammadi A, Sahebkar A, Iranshahi M, Amini M, Khojasteh R, Ghayour-Mobarhan M *et al*. Effects of supplementation with curcuminoids on dyslipidemia in obese patients: a randomized crossover trial. *Phytother Res*. 2013;27(3):374–9.

Mori A, Kabuto H, Pei YQ. Effects of piperine on convulsions and on brain serotonin and catecholamine levels in E1 mice. *Neurochem Res*. 1985;10(9):1269–75.

Mueller M, Beck V, Jungbauer A. PPARα activation by culinary herbs and spices. *Planta Med*. 2011;77(5):497–504.

Mujumdar AM, Dhuley JN, Deshmukh VK, Raman PH, Naik SR. Antiinflammatory activity of piperine. *Jpn J Med Sci Biol*. 1990;43(3):95–100.

Muralidhara, Narasimhamurthy K. Lack of genotoxic effects of piperine (the active principle of black pepper) in albino mice. *J Food Safety*. 1990;11(1):39–48.

Murthy CT, Bhattacharya S. Cryogenic grinding of black pepper. *J Food Eng*. 2008;85(1):18–28.

Murunikkara V, Pragasam SJ, Kodandaraman G, Sabina EP, Rasool M. Anti-inflammatory effect of piperine in adjuvant-induced arthritic rats a biochemical approach. *Inflammation*. 2012;35(4):1348–56.

Naidu KA, Thippeswamy NB. Inhibition of human low-density lipoprotein oxidation by active principles from spices. *Mol Cell Biochem*. 2002;229(1–2):19–23.

Narsimhan S. Plants and human civilization: Indian spices. *Comp Civiliz Rev*. 2009;60:120–48.

Nilani P, Kasthuribai N, Duraisamy B, Dhamodaran P, Ravichandran S, Ilango K *et al*. *In vitro* antioxidant activity of selected antiasthmatic herbal constituents. *Anc Sci Life*. 2009;28(4):3–6.

Nino. Getting pep in the kitchen (2007). Available at: http://www.houmatoday.com/news/20071017/getting-pep-in-the-kitchen. Accessed on: 16 November 2016.

Nogara L, Naber N, Pate E, Canton M, Reggiani C, Cooke R. Piperine's mitigation of obesity and diabetes can be explained by its up-regulation of the metabolic rate of resting muscle. *Proc Natl Acad Sci*. 2016;113(46):13009–14.

Ochiai A, Miyata S, Shimizu M, Inoue J, Sato R. Piperine induces hepatic low-density lipoprotein receptor expression through proteolytic activation of sterol regulatory element-binding proteins. *PLoS One*. 2015. DOI: 10.1371/journal.pone.0139799.

Ohtani M, Sugita M, Maruyama K. Amino acid mixture improves training efficiency in athletes. *J Nutr*. 2006;136(2):538S–43S.

REFERENCES

Okumura Y, Narukawa M, Watanabe T. Adiposity suppression effect in mice due to black pepper and its main pungent component, piperine. *Biosci Biotechnol Biochem*. 2010;74(8):1545–9.

Ouyang DY, Zeng LH, Pan H, Xu LH, Wang Y, Liu KP et al. Piperine inhibits the proliferation of human prostate cancer cells via induction of cell cycle arrest and autophagy. *Food Chem Toxicol*. 2013;60:424–30.

Paarakh PM, Sreeram DC, D SS, Ganapathy SP. *In vitro* cytotoxic and *in silico* activity of piperine isolated from *Piper nigrum* fruits Linn. *In Silico Pharmacol*. 2015. DOI: 10.1186/s40203-015-0013-2.

Panahi Y, Rahimnia AR, Sharafi M, Alishiri G, Saburi A, Sahebkar A. Curcuminoid treatment for knee osteoarthritis: a randomized double-blind placebo-controlled trial. *Phytother Res*. 2014;28(11):1625–31.

Panahi Y, Badeli R, Karami GR, Sahebkar A. Investigation of the efficacy of adjunctive therapy with bioavailability-boosted curcuminoids in major depressive disorder. *Phytother Res*. 2015;29(1):17–21.

Panahi Y, Hosseini MS, Khalili N, Naimi E, Soflaei SS, Majeed M et al. Effects of supplementation with curcumin on serum adipokine concentrations: a randomized controlled trial. *Nutrition*. 2016a; 32(10):1116–22.

Panahi Y, Hosseini MS, Khalili N, Naimi E, Simental-Mendía LE, Majeed M et al. Effects of curcumin on serum cytokine concentrations in subjects with metabolic syndrome: a post-hoc analysis of a randomized controlled trial. *Biomed Pharmacother*. 2016b;82:578–82.

Panahi Y, Khalili N, Sahebi E, Namazi S, Karimian MS, Majeed M et al. Antioxidant effects of curcuminoids in patients with type 2 diabetes mellitus: a randomized controlled trial. *Inflammopharmacology*. 2017;25(1):25–31.

Pany S, Pal A, Sahu PK. Potential neuroprotective effect of piperine in pilocarpine-induced temporal lobe epilepsy. *Indo Am J Pharm Res*. 2016;6(2):4369–75.

Park UH, Jeong HS, Jo EY, Park T, Yoon SK, Kim EJ et al. Piperine, a component of black pepper, inhibits adipogenesis by antagonizing PPARγ activity in 3T3L1 cells. *J Agric Food Chem*. 2012;60(15):3853–60.

Pathak N, Khandelwal S. Cytoprotective and immunomodulating properties of piperine on murine splenocytes: an *in vitro* study. *Eur J Pharmacol*. 2007;576(1–3):160–70.

Pathak N, Khandelwal S. Comparative efficacy of piperine, curcumin and Picroliv® against Cd immunotoxicity in mice. *Biometals*. 2008;21(6):649–61.

Patial V, S M, Sharma S, Pratap K, Singh D, Padwad YS. Synergistic effect of curcumin and piperine in suppression of DENA-induced hepatocellular carcinoma in rats. *Environ Toxicol Pharmacol*. 2015;40(2):445–52.

Patil VM, Das S, Balasubramanian K. Quantum chemical and docking insights into bioavailability enhancement of curcumin by piperine in pepper. *J Phys Chem A*. 2016;120(20):3643–53.

Pedersen BK. Exercise and cytokines. *Immunol Cell Biol*. 2000;78:532–5.

Peternelj TT, Coombes JS. Antioxidant supplementation during exercise training: beneficial or detrimental? *Sports Med*. 2011;41(12):1043–69.

REFERENCES

Pfund LY, Chamberlin BL and Matzger AJ. The bioenhancer piperine is at least trimorphic. *Cryst Growth Des.* 2015;15(5):2047–51.

Pingitore A, Lima GP, Mastorci F, Quinones A, Iervasi G, Vassalle C. Exercise and oxidative stress: potential effects of antioxidant dietary strategies in sports. *Nutrition.* 2015;31(7–8):916–22.

Piyachaturawat P, Glinsukon T, Toskulkao C. Acute and subacute toxicity of piperine in mice, rats and hamsters. *Toxicol Lett.* 1983;16(3–4):351–9.

Piyachaturawat P, Kingkaeohoi S, Toskulkao C. Potentiation of carbon tetrachloride hepatotoxicity by piperine. *Drug Chem Toxicol.* 1995;18(4):333–44.

Platel K, Srinivasan K. Influence of dietary spices or their active principles on digestive enzymes of small intestinal mucosa in rats. *Int J Food Sci Nutr.* 1996;47(1):55–9.

Platel K, Srinivasan K. Influence of dietary spices and their active principles on pancreatic digestive enzymes in albino rats. *Nahrung.* 2000;44(1):42–6.

Platel K, Srinivasan K. Studies on the influence of dietary spices on food transit time in experimental rats. *Nutr Res.* 2001;21(9):1309–14.

Platel K, Srinivasan K. Digestive stimulant action of spices: a myth or reality? *Indian J Med Res.* 2004;119(5):167–79.

Polley KR, Jenkins N, O'Connor P, McCully K. Influence of exercise training with resveratrol supplementation on skeletal muscle mitochondrial capacity. *Appl Physiol Nutr Metab.* 2016;41(1):26–32.

Popovich DG, Yeo CR, Zhang W. Ginsenosides derived from Asian (*Panax ginseng*), American Ginseng (*Panax quinquefolius*) and potential cytoactivity. *Int J Biomed Pharm Sci.* 2012;6(1):56–62.

Pradeep CR, Kuttan G. Effect of piperine on the inhibition of lung metastasis-induced B16F10 melanoma cells in mice. *Clin Exp Metastasis.* 2002;19(8):703–8.

Pradeep CR, Kuttan G. Effect of piperine on the inhibition of nitric oxide (NO) and TNF-alpha production. *Immunopharmacol Immunotoxicol.* 2003;25(3):337–46.

Pradeep CR, Kuttan G. Piperine is a potent inhibitor of nuclear factor-kappaB (NF-kappaB), c-Fos, CREB, ATF2 and proinflammatory cytokine gene expression in B16F10 melanoma cells. *Int Immunopharmacol.* 2004;4(14):1795–803.

Prakash UN, Srinivasan K. Beneficial influence of dietary spices on the ultrastructure and fluidity of the intestinal brush border in rats. *Br J Nutr.* 2010;104(1):31–9.

Prakash UN, Srinivasan K. Enhanced intestinal uptake of iron, zinc and calcium in rats fed pungent spice principles--piperine, capsaicin and ginger (*Zingiber officinale*). *J Trace Elem Med Biol.* 2013;27(3):184–90.

Prasad NS, Raghavendra R, Lokesh BR, Naidu KA. Spice phenolics inhibit human PMNL 5-lipoxygenase. *Prostaglandins Leukot Essent Fatty Acids.* 2004;70(6):521–8.

REFERENCES

Rabbani SA, Ali SM. Effect of piperine on pentylenetetrazole-induced seizures, cognition and oxidative stress in mice. Afr J Pharm Pharmacol. 2015;9(12):433–9.

Randhawa GK, Kullar JS, Rajkumar. Bioenhancers from mother nature and their applicability in modern medicine. Int J Appl Basic Med Res. 2011;1(1):5–10.

Rauscher FM, Sanders RA, Watkins JB 3rd. Effects of piperine on antioxidant pathways in tissues from normal and streptozotoc-ininduced diabetic rats. J Biochem Mol Toxicol. 2000;14(6):329–34.

Ravindran PN. Introduction. In: Ravindran PN (Ed). Black pepper: *Piper nigrum*. Medicinal and Aromatic Plants — Industrial Profiles. Amsterdam: Harwood Academic Publishers; 2000. p. 1–9.

Rawlinson HG. From the earliest times of the fall of Babylon. In: Intercourse between India and the western world: From the earliest times of the fall of Rome. New Delhi: Asian Educational Services; 2002. p. 14.

Reddy AC, Lokesh BR. Studies on spice principles as antioxidants in the inhibition of lipid peroxidation of rat liver microsomes. Mol Cell Biochem. 1992;111(1–2):117–24.

Reen RK, Jamwal DS, Taneja SC, Koul JL, Dubey RK, Wiebel FJ et al. Impairment of UDP-glucose dehydrogenase and glucuronidation activities in liver and small intestine of rat and guinea pig in vitro by piperine. Biochem Pharmacol. 1993;46(2):229–38.

Reen RK, Roesch SF, Kiefer F, Wiebel FJ, Singh J. Piperine impairs cytochrome P4501A1 activity by direct interaction with the enzyme and not by downregulation of CYP1A1 gene expression in the rat hepatoma 5L cell line. Biochem Biophys Res Commun. 1996;218(2):562–9.

Rehman A, Mehmood MH, Haneef M, Gilani AH, Ilyas M, Siddiqui BS et al. Potential of black pepper as a functional food for treatment of airways disorders. J Funct Foods. 2015;19:126–140.

Rinwa P, Kumar A. Piperine potentiates the protective effects of curcumin against chronic unpredictable stress-induced cognitive impairment and oxidative damage in mice. Brain Res. 2012;1488:38–50.

Rinwa P, Kumar A, Garg S. Suppression of neuroinflammatory and apoptotic signaling cascade by curcumin alone and in combination with piperine in rat model of olfactory bulbectomy-induced depression. PLoS One. 2013. DOI: 10.1371/journal.pone.0061052.

Rinwa P, Kumar A. Quercetin along with piperine prevents cognitive dysfunction, oxidative stress and neuro-inflammation associated with mouse model of chronic unpredictable stress. Arch Pharm Res. 2013. DOI: 10.1007/s12272-013-0205-4.

Roberts CK, Hevener AL, Barnard RJ. Metabolic syndrome and insulin resistance: underlying causes and modification by exercise training. Compr Physiol. 2013;3(1):1–58.

Rodgers G, Doucette CD, Soutar DA, Liwski RS, Hoskin DW. Piperine impairs the migration and T cell-activating function of dendritic cells. Toxicol Lett. 2016;242:23–33.

REFERENCES

Rogerio AP, Carlo T, Ambrosio SR. Bioactive natural molecules and traditional herbal medicine in the treatment of airways diseases. *Evid Based Complement Alternat Med*. 2016. DOI: 10.1155/2016/9872302.

Rondanelli M, Opizzi A, Perna S, Faliva M, Solerte SB, Fioravanti M *et al*. Improvement in insulin resistance and favourable changes in plasma inflammatory adipokines after weight loss associated with two months' consumption of a combination of bioactive food ingredients in overweight subjects. *Endocrine*. 2013;44(2):391–401.

Rosenbaum T, Simon SA. TRPV1 Receptors and Signal Transduction. In: Liedtke WB, Heller S (Eds). TRP Ion Channel Function in Sensory Transduction and Cellular Signaling Cascades. Boca Raton (FL): CRC Press Taylor and Francis; 2007.

Ryu EK, Choe YS, Lee KH, Choi Y, Kim BT. Curcumin and dehydrozingerone derivatives: synthesis, radiolabeling, and evaluation for beta-amyloid plaque imaging. *J Med Chem*. 2006;49(20):6111–9.

Sabina EP, Nagar S, Rasool M. A role of piperine on monosodium urate crystal-induced inflammation – an experimental model of gouty arthritis. *Inflammation*. 2011;34(3):184–92.

Sama V, Nadipelli M, Yenumula P, Bommineni MR, Mullangi R. Effect of piperine on antihyperglycemic activity and pharmacokinetic profile of nateglinide. *Arzneimittelforschung*. 2012;62(8):384–8.

Samra YA, Said HS, Elsherbiny NM, Liou GI, El-Shishtawy MM, Eissa LA. Cepharanthine and piperine ameliorate diabetic nephropathy in rats: role of NF-κB and NLRP3 inflammasome. *Life Sci*. 2016;157:187–99.

Samykutty A, Shetty AV, Dakshinamoorthy G, Bartik MM, Johnson GL, Webb B *et al*. Piperine, a bioactive component of pepper spice exerts therapeutic effects on androgen dependent and androgen independent prostate cancer cells. *PLoS One*. 2013. DOI: 10.1372/journal.pone.0065889.

Santini A, Tenore GC, Novellino E. Nutraceuticals: a paradigm of proactive medicine. *Eur J Pharm Sci*. 2017;96:53–61.

Saraogi P, Vohora D, Khanam R, Pillai KK. Combination therapy of piperine and phenytoin in maximal electroshock-induced seizures in mice: isobolographic and biochemical analysis. *Drug Res*. 2013;63(6):311–8.

Scott IM, Jensen HR, Philogène BJR, Arnason JT. A review of Piper spp. (Piperaceae) phytochemistry, insecticidal activity and mode of action. *Phytochem Rev*. 2008;7:65–75.

Selvendiran K, Singh JP, Krishnan KB, Sakthisekaran D. Cytoprotective effect of piperine against benzo[a]pyrene-induced lung cancer with reference to lipid peroxidation and antioxidant system in Swiss albino mice. *Fitoterapia*. 2003;74(1–2):109–15.

Selvendiran K, Sakthisekaran D. Chemopreventive effect of piperine on modulating lipid peroxidation and membrane bound enzymes in benzo(a)pyrene-induced lung carcinogenesis. *Biomed Pharmacother*. 2004;58(4):264–7.

REFERENCES

Selvendiran K, Senthilnathan P, Magesh V, Sakthisekaran D. Modulatory effect of piperine on mitochondrial antioxidant system in benzo(a)pyrene-induced experimental lung carcinogenesis. *Phytomedicine*. 2004a;11(1):85–9.

Selvendiran K, Banu SM, Sakthisekaran D. Protective effect of piperine on benzo(a)pyrene-induced lung carcinogenesis in Swiss albino mice. *Clin Chim Acta*. 2004b;350(1–2):73–8.

Selvendiran K, Thirunavukkarasu C, Singh JP, Padmavathi R, Sakthisekaran D. Chemopreventive effect of piperine on mitochondrial TCA cycle and phase I and glutathione metabolizing enzymes in benzo(a)pyrene-induced lung carcinogenesis in Swiss albino mice. *Mol Cell Biochem*. 2005a;271(1–2):101–6.

Selvendiran K, Banu SM, Sakthisekaran D. Oral supplementation of piperine leads to altered phase II enzymes and reduced DNA damage and DNA protein cross links in benzo(a)pyrene-induced experimental lung carcinogenesis. *Mol Cell Biochem*. 2005b;268(1–2):141–7.

Selvendiran K, Padmavathi R, Magesh V, Sakthisekaran D. Preliminary study on inhibition of genotoxicity by piperine in mice. *Fitoterapia*. 2005c;76(3–4):296–300.

Selvendiran K, Prince Vijeya Singh J, Sakthisekaran D. *In vivo* effect of piperine on serum and tissue glycoprotein levels in benzo(a)pyrene-induced lung carcinogenesis in Swiss albino mice. *Pulm Pharmacol Ther*. 2006;19(2):107–11.

Shaffer M. Meet the Pipers. In: Pepper—A History of the World's Most Influential Spice. New York: Thomas Dunne Books; 2013. p. 1–2.

Shah S, Shah G, Patel M, Singh S. Effect of piperine in obesity-induced insulin resistance and type-II diabetes mellitus in rats. *J Nat Rem*. 2010;10(2):116–22.

Shoba G, Joy D, Joseph T, Majeed M, Rajendran R, Srinivas PS. Influence of piperine on the pharmacokinetics of curcumin in animals and human volunteers. *Planta Med*. 1998;64(4):353–6.

Singh J, Dubey RK, Atal CK. Piperine-mediated inhibition of glucuronidation activity in isolated epithelial cells of the guinea-pig small intestine: evidence that piperine lowers the endogenous UDP-glucuronic acid content. *J Pharmacol Exp Ther*. 1986;236(2):488–93.

Singh J, Reen RK, Wiebel FJ. Piperine, a major ingredient of black and long peppers, protects against AFB1-induced cytotoxicity and micronuclei formation in H4IIEC3 rat hepatoma cells. *Cancer Lett*. 1994;86(2):195–200.

Singh R, Singh N, Saini BS, Rao HS. *In vitro* antioxidant activity of pet ether extract of black pepper. *Indian J Pharmacol*. 2008;40(4):147–51.

Singh S, Jamwal S, Kumar P. Piperine enhances the protective effect of curcumin against 3-NP-induced neurotoxicity: possible neurotransmitters modulation mechanism. *Neurochem Res*. 2015;40(8):1758–66.

Singh S, Kumar P. Neuroprotective activity of curcumin in combination with piperine against quinolinic acid-induced neurodegeneration in rats. *Pharmacology*. 2016;97(3–4):151–60.

REFERENCES

Singh S, Kumar P. Neuroprotective potential of curcumin in combination with piperine against 6-hydroxy dopamine induced motor deficit and neurochemical alterations in rats. *Inflammopharmacology.* 2017;25:69–79.

Solecki RS. Shanidar IV, a Neanderthal flower burial in northern Iraq. *Science.* 1975;190(4217):880–1.

Song XY, Xu S, Hu JF, Tang J, Chu SF, Liu H et al. Piperine prevents cholesterol gallstones formation in mice. *Eur J Pharmacol.* 2015;751:112–7.

Srinivasan K. Black pepper (*Piper nigrum*) and Its Bioactive Compound, Piperine. In: Aggarwal BB, Kunnumakkara AB (Eds). Molecular Targets and Therapeutic Uses of Spices: Modern Uses for Ancient Medicine. Ames: World Scientific Publishing Co. Inc; 2009. p. 25–64.

Srinivasan K. Black pepper and its pungent principle-piperine: a review of diverse physiological effects. *Crit Rev Food Sci Nutr.* 2007;47(8):735–48.

Srinivasan MR, Satyanarayana MN. Effect of black pepper (*Piper nigrum* Linn) and piperine on growth, blood constituents and organ weight in rats. *Nutr Rep Int.* 1981;23(5):871–6.

Sruthi D, Zachariah TJ, Leela NK, Jayarajan K. Correlation between chemical profiles of black pepper (*Piper nigrum* L.) var. Panniyur-1 collected from different locations. *J Med Plants Res.* 2013;7(31):2349–57.

Suresh D, Srinivasan K. Studies on the *in vitro* absorption of spice principles – curcumin, capsaicin and piperine in rat intestines. *Food Chem Toxicol.* 2007a;45(8):1437–42.

Suresh DV, Mahesha HG, Rao AG, Srinivasan K. Binding of bioactive phytochemical piperine with human serum albumin: a spectrofluorometric study. *Biopolymers.* 2007b;86(4):265–75.

Suresh D, Srinivasan K. Tissue distribution & elimination of capsaicin, piperine & curcumin following oral intake in rats. *Indian J Med Res.* 2010;131:682–91.

Tabatabaei-Malazy O, Larijani B, Abdollahi M. Targeting metabolic disorders by natural products. *J Diabetes Metab Disord.* 2015. DOI: 10.1186/s40200-015-0184-8.

Tak JK, Lee JH, Park JW. Resveratrol and piperine enhance radiosensitivity of tumor cells. *BMB Rep.* 2012;45(4):242–6.

Takeuchi K, Ueshima K, Ohuchi T, Okabe S. The role of capsaicin-sensitive sensory neurons in healing of HCl-induced gastric mucosal lesions in rats. *Gastroenterology.* 1994;106(6):1524–32.

Taqvi SI, Shah AJ, Gilani AH. Blood pressure lowering and vasomodulator effects of piperine. *J Cardiovasc Pharmacol.* 2008;52(5):452–8.

Tasleem F, Azhar I, Ali SN, Perveen S, Mahmood ZA. Analgesic and anti-inflammatory activities of *Piper nigrum* L. *Asian Pac J Trop Med.* 2014. DOI: 10.1016/S1995-7645(14)60275-3.

REFERENCES

Tharmalingam N, Kim SH, Park M, Woo HJ, Kim HW, Yang JY et al. Inhibitory effect of piperine on *Helicobacter pylori* growth and adhesion to gastric adenocarcinoma cells. *Infect Agent Cancer*. 2014. DOI: 101186/1750-9378-9-43.

Tharmalingam N, Park M, Lee MH, Woo HJ, Kim HW, Yang JY et al. Piperine treatment suppresses *Helicobacter pylori* toxin entry in to gastric epithelium and minimizes β-catenin-mediated oncogenesis and IL-8 secretion *in vitro*. *Am J Transl Res*. 2016;8(2):885–98.

Thiel A, Buskens C, Woehrle T, Etheve S, Schoenmakers A, Fehr M et al. Black pepper constituent piperine: genotoxicity studies *in vitro* and *in vivo*. *Food Chem Toxicol*. 2014;66:350–7.

Toussaint-Samat M (Translated by: Bell A). Spice at any price. In: A History of Food. West Sussex: Willey-Blackwell; 2009. p. 443.

Tu Y, Sun D, Zeng X, Yao N, Huang X, Huang D et al. Piperine potentiates the hypocholesterolemic effect of curcumin in rats fed on a high-fat diet. *Exp Ther Med*. 2014;8(1):260–6.

Tunsophon S, Chootip K. Comparative effects of piperine and simvastatin in fat accumulation and antioxidative status in high-fat-induced hyperlipidemic rats. *Can J Physiol Pharmacol*. 2016;94(12):1344–8.

Umar S, Golam Sarwar AH, Umar K, Ahmad N, Sajad M, Ahmad S et al. Piperine ameliorates oxidative stress, inflammation and histological outcome in collagen induced arthritis. *Cell Immunol*. 2013;284(1–2):51–9.

Vazquez-Olivencia W, Shah P, Pitchumoni CS. The effect of red and black pepper on orocecal transit time. *J Am Coll Nutr*. 1992;11(2):228–31.

Veeresham C, Sujatha S, Rani TS. Effect of piperine on the pharmacokinetics and pharmacodynamics of glimepiride in normal and streptozotocin-induced diabetic rats. *Nat Prod Commun*. 2012;7(10):1283–6.

Vijayakumar RS, Nalini N. Piperine, an active principle from *Piper nigrum*, modulates hormonal and apo lipoprotein profiles in hyperlipidemic rats. *J Basic Clin Physiol Pharmacol*. 2006a;17(2):71–86.

Vijayakumar RS, Nalini N. Efficacy of piperine, an alkaloidal constituent from *Piper nigrum* on erythrocyte antioxidant status in high-fat diet and antithyroid drug induced hyperlipidemic rats. *Cell Biochem Funct*. 2006b;24(6):491–8.

Vijayakumar RS, Surya D, Nalini N. Antioxidant efficacy of black pepper (*Piper nigrum* L.) and piperine in rats with high-fat diet-induced oxidative stress. *Redox Rep*. 2004;9(2):105–10.

Volak LP, Hanley MJ, Masse G, Hazarika S, Harmatz JS, Badmaev V et al. Effect of a herbal extract containing curcumin and piperine on midazolam, flurbiprofen and paracetamol (acetaminophen) pharmacokinetics in healthy volunteers. *Br J Clin Pharmacol*. 2013;75(2):450–62.

Wadhwa S, Singhal S, Rawat S. Bioavailability enhancement by piperine: a review. *Asian J Biomed Pharm Sci*. 2014;36(4):1–8.

REFERENCES

Walter AA, Herda TJ, Ryan ED, Costa PB, Hoge KM, Beck TW et al. Acute effects of a thermogenic nutritional supplement on cycling time to exhaustion and muscular strength in college-aged men. *J Int Soc Sports Nutr.* 2009. DOI: 10.1186/1550-2783-6-15.

Wattanathorn J, Chonpathompikunlert P, Muchimapura S, Priprem A, Tankamnerdthai O. Piperine, the potential functional food for mood and cognitive disorders. *Food Chem Toxicol.* 2008;46(9):3106–10.

Westerterp-Plantenga M, Diepvens K, Joosen AM, Bérubé-Parent S, Tremblay A. Metabolic effects of spices, teas, and caffeine. *Physiol Behav.* 2006;89(1):85–91.

White PA, Oliveira RC, Oliveira AP, Serafini MR, Araújo AA, Gelain DP et al. Antioxidant activity and mechanisms of action of natural compounds isolated from lichens: a systematic review. *Molecules.* 2014;19(9):14496–527.

Wightman EL, Reay JL, Haskell CF, Williamson G, Dew TP, Kennedy DO. Effects of resveratrol alone or in combination with piperine on cerebral blood flow parameters and cognitive performance in human subjects: a randomised, double-blind, placebo-controlled, cross-over investigation. *Br J Nutr.* 2014;112(2):203–13.

Williams M. Dietary supplements and sports performance: amino acids. *J Int Soc Sports Nutr.* 2005;2(2):63–7.

Williams M. Dietary supplements and sports performance: herbals. *J Int Soc Sports Nutr.* 2006;3:1–6.

Williams MH. Dietary supplements and sports performance: introduction and vitamins. *J Int Soc Sports Nutr.* 2004;1:1–6.

Williams AR, Ramsay A, Hansen TVA, Ropiak HM, Mejer H, Nejsum P et al. Anthelmintic activity of *trans*-cinnamaldehyde and A- and B-type proanthocyanidins derived from cinnamon (*Cinnamomum verum*). *Sci Rep.* 2015. DOI: 10.1038/srep14791.

Wittchen HU, Jacobi F, Rehm J, Gustavsson A, Svensson M, Jönsson B et al. The size and burden of mental disorders and other disorders of the brain in Europe 2010. *Eur Neuropsychopharmacol.* 2011;21(9):655–79.

Wongpa S, Himakoun L, Soontornchai S, Temcharoen P. Antimutagenic effects of piperine on cyclophosphamide-induced chromosome aberrations in rat bone marrow cells. *Asian Pac J Cancer Prev.* 2007;8(4):623–7.

Woo HM, Kang JH, Kawada T, Yoo H, Sung MK, Yu R. Active spice-derived components can inhibit inflammatory responses of adipose tissue in obesity by suppressing inflammatory actions of macrophages and release of monocyte chemoattractant protein1 from adipocytes. *Life Sci.* 2007;80(10):926–31.

Xia Y, Khoi PN, Yoon HJ, Lian S, Joo YE, Chay KO et al. Piperine inhibits IL-1β-induced IL6 expression by suppressing p38 MAPK and STAT3 activation in gastric cancer cells. *Mol Cell Biochem.* 2015;398(1–2):147–56.

Xu Y, Zhang C, Wu F, Xu X, Wang G, Lin M et al. Piperine potentiates the effects of *trans*-resveratrol on stress-induced depressive-like behavior: involvement of monoaminergic system and cAMP-dependent pathway. *Metab Brain Dis.* 2016;31(4):837–48.

REFERENCES

Yaffe PB, Doucette CD, Walsh M, Hoskin DW. Piperine impairs cell cycle progression and causes reactive oxygen species-dependent apoptosis in rectal cancer cells. *Exp Mol Pathol*. 2013;94(1):109–14.

Yaffe PB, Power Coombs MR, Doucette CD, Walsh M, Hoskin DW. Piperine, an alkaloid from black pepper, inhibits growth of human colon cancer cells via G1 arrest and apoptosis triggered by endoplasmic reticulum stress. *Mol Carcinog*. 2015;54(10):1070–85.

Yang W, Chen YH, Liu H, Qu HD. Neuroprotective effects of piperine on the 1-methyl-4-phenyl-1,2,3,6-tetrahydropyridine-induced Parkinson's disease mouse model. *Int J Mol Med*. 2015;36(5):1369–76.

Ying X, Chen X, Cheng S, Shen Y, Peng L, Xu HZ. Piperine inhibits IL-β induced expression of inflammatory mediators in human osteoarthritis chondrocyte. *Int Immunopharmacol*. 2013a;17(2):293–9.

Ying X, Yu K, Chen X, Chen H, Hong J, Cheng S et al. Piperine inhibits LPS induced expression of inflammatory mediators in RAW 264.7 cells. *Cell Immunol*. 2013b;285(1–2):49–54.

Zeng X, Cai D, Zeng Q, Chen Z, Zhong G, Zhuo J et al. Selective reduction in the expression of UGTs and SULTs, a novel mechanism by which piperine enhances the bioavailability of curcumin in rat. *Biopharm Drug Dispos*. 2017;38(1):3–19.

Zhai WJ, Zhang ZB, Xu NN, Guo YF, Qiu C, Li C et al. Piperine plays an anti-inflammatory role in *Staphylococcus aureus* endometritis by inhibiting activation of NF-κB and MAPK pathways in mice. *Evid Based Complement Alternat Med*. 2016. DOI: 10.1155/2016/8597208.

Zhang J, Zhu X, Li H, Li B, Sun L, Xie T et al. Piperine inhibits proliferation of human osteosarcoma cells via G2/M phase arrest and metastasis by suppressing MMP2/9 expression. *Int Immunopharmacol*. 2015;24(1):50–8.

Zhang W, Han Y, Lim SL, Lim LY. Dietary regulation of P-gp function and expression. *Expert Opin Drug Metab Toxicol*. 2009;5(7):789–801.

Zhou S, Lim LY, Chowbay B. Herbal modulation of P-glycoprotein. *Drug Metab Rev*. 2004;36(1):57–104.

Glossary

3-NP

3-Nitropropionic acid: A toxin produced by certain plants and fungi. It has been used to produce an animal model for study of Huntington's disease, a neurodegenerative disorder.

3-OH-BAP

3-Hydroxy-Benzo(a)pyrene: A metabolite of benzo(a)pyrene (BAP), a common environmental pollutant and a potent carcinogen.

5-HT

5-Hydroxytryptamine/Serotonin: A monoamine neurotransmitter, popularly thought to be a contributor to feelings of well being and happiness.

ABTS

2,2'-Azino-bis(3-ethylbenzothiazoline-6-sulphonic acid): A peroxidase substrate used to observe the reaction kinetics of specific enzymes. A common use for it is in the enzyme-linked immunosorbent assay (ELISA) to detect for binding of molecules to each other.

AChE

Acetylcholinesterase: An enzyme that catalyzes the breakdown of acetylcholine and some other choline esters that function as neurotransmitters.

ADAMTS

A Disintegrin And Metalloproteinase with Thrombospondin motifs: A family of multidomain extracellular protease enzymes and are the key enzymes of the extracellular matrix.

AHH

Aryl Hydrocarbon Hydroxylase: A multi-component, microsomal-bound enzyme system, which eliminates a number of lipid-soluble compounds from the body by converting them into water-soluble forms.

ANS

Autonomous Nervous System: A division of central nervous system that regulates bodily functions, such as the heart rate, digestion, respiratory rate, pupillary response, urination etc.

AP-1

Activator Protein 1: A transcription factor that regulates gene expression in response to a variety of stimuli, including cytokines, growth factors, stress and bacterial and viral infections.

Apo

Apolipoproteins: These are proteins that bind to lipids to form lipoproteins, whose main function is to transport lipids.

GLOSSARY

ATP
Adenosine Triphosphate: An energy-carrying molecule found in the body cells. It carries chemical energy obtained from the breakdown of food molecules and releases it to fuel other cellular processes.

AUC
Area Under Curve: It reflects the concentration of drug in blood plasma and actual body exposure to drug after administration.

Aβ
Amyloid Beta: The peptides of 36–43 amino acids that are majorly involved in Alzheimer's disease as the main component of the amyloid plaques found in the brain of Alzheimer's patients.

BALF
Bronchoalveolar Lavage Fluid: It is the fluid squirted into a small part of the lung and then collected for examination, diagnosis of disease or evaluation of treatment.

BAP
Benzo(a)pyrene: A potent mutagen and carcinogen produced during incomplete combustion of organic compounds such as oil, gasoline and charbroiled food.

BCAAs
Branched Chain Amino Acids: Amino acids having aliphatic side-chains with a branch (e.g. leucine, isoleucine and valine), an essential nutrient that is obtained from proteins found in food, especially meat, dairy products, and legumes.

BCE
Before the Common (or Current) Era: It denotes the same numeric values as the Anno Domini (AD) year-numbering system introduced by the 6th century Christian monk Dionysius Exiguus, intending the beginning of the life of Jesus to be the reference date.

BDNF
Brain-derived Neurotrophic Factor: A protein, member of the neurotrophin family of growth factors, helps to support the survival of existing neurons and encourage the growth and differentiation of new neurons and synapses.

BHA
Butylated Hydroxyanisole: An antioxidant used as a food preservative in food, food packaging, animal feed, cosmetics, rubber, and petroleum products.

BHT
Butylated Hydroxytoluene: A lipophilic organic compound used as a preservative in food and personal care products.

BMDCs
Bone Marrow-derived Dendritic Cells: Antigen-presenting cells derived from the bone marrow, which act as messengers between the innate and the adaptive immune systems.

BMI
Body Mass Index: A measure of body fat, derived from the mass (weight) and height of an individual.

GLOSSARY

BP
Blood Pressure: It is the pressure of circulating blood on the walls of blood vessels. When used without further specification, "blood pressure" usually refers to the arterial pressure in the systemic circulation.

cAMP
cyclic Adenosine Monophosphate: A derivative of ATP, acts as a second messenger in many biological processes for intracellular signal transduction in many different organisms, conveying the cAMP-dependent pathway.

CBF
Cerebral Blood Flow: It is defined as the volume of blood passing through a given amount of brain tissue per unit of time.

CCl_4
Carbon Tetrachloride: An organic compound widely used as an animal model by administering to rodents to study mechanisms of hepatic injury.

CE
Common (or Current) Era: It denotes the same numeric values as the Anno Domini (AD) year-numbering system introduced by the 6th century Christian monk Dionysius Exiguus, intending the beginning of the life of Jesus to be the reference date.

CFA
Complete Freund's Adjuvant: A solution of antigen emulsified in mineral oil composed of inactivated and dried mycobacteria. It is effective in stimulating cell-mediated immunity and leads to potentiation T helper cells that lead to the production of certain immunoglobulins and effector T cells.

C_{max}
Concentration Maximum: A term used in pharmacokinetics refers to the maximum (or peak) serum concentration that a drug achieves in a specified compartment or test area of the body after its administration.

CMS
Chronic Mild Stress: An animal model of depression that aims to mimic a chronic depressive-like state that develops gradually over time in response to stress.

CNS
Central Nervous System: The part of the nervous system consisting of the brain and spinal cord. It integrates information it receives from, and coordinates and influences the activity of all parts of the body.

CoQ10
Coenzyme Q10: A coenzyme that is ubiquitously present in most animals, primarily in the mitochondria. It participates in aerobic cellular respiration, which generates energy in the form of ATP.

COX-2
Cyclooxygenase-2: An enzyme that plays a major role in pain and inflammation.

CRP
C-reactive Protein: A protein found in blood plasma, produced by the liver. It is a marker of inflammation.

GLOSSARY

CUS
Chronic Unpredictable Stress: An animal model of human depression, wherein after prolonged exposure of tested animals to a series of unpredictable mild stressors, a condition similar to anhedonia develops, which is observed in the majority of depressive disorders.

CYP2C9
Cytochrome P450 2C9: An important cytochrome P450 enzyme with a major role in the oxidation of both xenobiotic and endogenous compounds.

CYP3A4
Cytochrome P450 3A4: A member of the cytochrome P450 family of oxidizing enzymes, mainly found in the liver and in the intestine. It helps remove xenobiotics, such as toxins or drugs from the body by the process of oxidation.

CYP7A1
Cholesterol 7α-hydroxylase: A liver-specific enzyme that catalyzes the 7α-hydroxylation of cholesterol, the limiting step in the classical pathway responsible for the conversion of cholesterol into bile acids.

DENA
Diethylnitrosamine: A chemical carcinogen with the potential to cause tumors in various organs, including the liver, skin, gastrointestinal tract and respiratory system.

DEX
Dexamethasone: A corticosteroid used to treat a number of different conditions, such as inflammation, severe allergies, adrenal problems, arthritis, asthma etc.

DNA
Deoxyribonucleic Acid: A molecule that carries the genetic instructions used in the growth, development, functioning and reproduction of all known living organisms and many viruses.

DPPH
2-Diphenyl-1-Picrylhydrazyl: A dark-colored crystalline powder used as a monitor of chemical reactions involving radicals (e.g. antioxidant assay).

DRX
Disordered Relaxed State: One of the two resting states of skeletal muscle myosin, wherein it is disordered and moving freely in the inter-filament space.

DSHEA
Dietary Supplement Health and Education Act: A 1994 statute of the United States Federal Legislation, which defines and regulates dietary supplements.

EC_{50}
Half-maximal Effective Concentration: It is a quantitative measure that refers to the concentration of a drug, antibody or toxicant, which induces a response halfway between the baseline and maximum after a specified exposure time.

EGCG
Epigallocatechin-3-gallate: A type of catechin, most abundantly found in tea, and used in many dietary supplements.

GLOSSARY

ELISA

Enzyme-linked Immunosorbent Assay: A plate-based assay technique designed for detecting and quantifying substances such as peptides, proteins, antibodies and hormones.

ERK

Extracellular Signal-regulated Kinases: Widely expressed protein kinase intracellular signalling molecules that are activated by different stimuli, such as growth factors, cytokines, virus infection etc.

FACS

Fluorescence-activated Cell Sorting: A specialized type of flow cytometry that provides a method for sorting a population of cells into sub-populations based on fluorescent labelling.

FDA

Food and Drug Administration: A federal agency of the United States Department of Health and Human Services, which is responsible for protecting and promoting public health through the control and supervision of food safety, tobacco products, dietary supplements, prescription and over-the-counter drugs etc.

FLS

Fibroblast-like Synoviocytes: A specialised cell type located inside joints in the synovium, which plays a crucial role in the pathogenesis of chronic inflammatory diseases, such as rheumatoid arthritis.

FST

Forced Swim Test: A rodent behavioral test used for evaluation of antidepressant drugs, antidepressant efficacy of new compounds, and experimental manipulations that are aimed at rendering or preventing depressive-like states.

GABA

γ-Aminobutyric Acid: A chief inhibitory neurotransmitter in the mammalian central nervous system and is also directly responsible for the regulation of muscle tone. GABA is of pharmacological importance in the function of many anti-anxiety drugs as well.

GE

Gastric Emptying: A physiological process involving evacuation of food from the stomach into the duodenum.

GRAS

Generally Recognized As Safe: A regulatory designation first introduced by the USFDA under the Federal Food, Drug, and Cosmetic Act (the Act) for any substance that is generally recognized, among qualified experts, as having been adequately shown to be safe under the conditions of its intended use.

GSH

Glutathione: An important antioxidant capable of preventing damage to important cellular components caused by reactive oxygen species, such as free radicals.

GST

Glutathione-S-Transferase: A phase II metabolic isozyme that catalyzes the conjugation of the reduced form of glutathione to xenobiotic substrates for the purpose of detoxification.

GLOSSARY

GT
Gastrointestinal Transit: It is the time taken by food to leave the stomach and travel through the intestines.

H_2O_2
Hydrogen Peroxide: A strong oxidizing agent used in aqueous solution as a ripening agent, bleach, and topical anti-infective.

HDL
High-density Lipoproteins: One of the five major groups of lipoproteins, often referred to as "good" cholesterol as they help remove excess cholesterol from the body.

HFD
High-fat Diet: A diet rich in fat that promotes the development of obesity.

HOMA
Homeostatic Model Assessment: A method used to quantify insulin resistance and beta-cell function.

HPA Axis
Hypothalamic-Pituitary-Adrenal Axis: A complex set of direct influences and feedback interactions among three endocrine glands: the hypothalamus, the pituitary gland and the adrenal glands that controls reactions to stress and regulates many body processes.

HPLC
High-performance Liquid Chromatography: An analytical technique used to separate, identify and quantify each component in a mixture of compounds soluble in a particular solvent.

HPTLC
High-performance Thin-layer Chromatography: The most advanced form of TLC and comprises the use of chromatographic layers of utmost separation efficiency and the employment of state-of-the-art instrumentation for all steps in the procedure.

IC_{50}
Half-maximal Inhibitory Concentration: It is a quantitative measure of the effectiveness of a substance in inhibiting a specific biological or biochemical function by 50%.

IDD
Intervertebral Disc Degeneration: A condition of the discs between vertebrae with loss of cushioning, fragmentation and herniation related to aging.

IgE
Immunoglobulin E: A kind of antibody, whose main function is immune defense and plays a pivotal role in responses to allergens.

ILs
Interleukins: A type of cytokines, which play a very important role in nearly all aspects of inflammation and immunity.

iNOS
Inducible Nitric Oxide Synthase: A key enzyme generating nitric oxide that plays an important role in numerous physiological and pathological conditions.

GLOSSARY

IUPAC

International Union of Pure and Applied Chemistry: An international federation of National Adhering Organizations that represents chemists in individual countries, which has created a set of rules to generate systematic names for chemical compounds. These chemical nomenclatures are used most frequently worldwide.

IVDs

Intervertebral Discs: These are fibrocartilaginous cushions serving as the spine's shock absorbing system, which protect the vertebrae, brain, and other structures (i.e. nerves).

JECFA

The Joint FAO/WHO Expert Committee on Food Additives: An international expert scientific committee administered jointly by the Food and Agriculture Organization of the United Nations (FAO) and the World Health Organization (WHO). It serves as an independent scientific committee, which performs risk assessments and provides advice to FAO, WHO and the member countries of both organizations.

JNK

c-Jun N-terminal Kinases: A member of the mitogen-activated protein kinase (MAPK) family that regulates a range of biological processes.

K_i

Inhibitory Constant: An indication of how potent an inhibitor is. A function of the inhibitor concentration.

L-(+)-Selenomethionine (LSM):

It is the amino acid methionine with selenium substituting for the sulphur moiety. L(+)-selenomethionine is considered as a safe, efficacious and bioavailable form of selenium, which is an essential micronutrient for humans.

LCAT

Lecithin Cholesterol Acyl Transferase: A lipoprotein-associated enzyme, which plays a large role in the esterification of free cholesterol, the maturation of HDL particles and the intravascular stage of reverse cholesterol transport.

LD_{50}

Median Lethal Dose: It is the amount of an substance that kills 50 percent of the animals in a dose group.

LDL

Low-density Lipoprotein: A class of lipoprotein particles, which carry cholesterol in the blood and around the body, for use by cells. It is commonly referred to as "bad cholesterol" due to the link between high LDL levels and cardiovascular disease.

LDLR

Low-density Lipoprotein Receptor: A cell-surface receptor that mediates the endocytosis of cholesterol-rich LDL.

L-NAME

N(G)-Nitro-L-arginine Methyl Ester: An analog of arginine that inhibits nitric oxide production. It has multiple effects on the vascular system.

GLOSSARY

LPS

Lipopolysaccharide: The major component of the outer membrane of Gram-negative bacteria, known to cause distinct depressive-like behavioral syndrome when administered to rodents.

LXR

Liver X Receptor: A member of the nuclear receptor family of transcription factors, which are important regulators of cholesterol, fatty acid and glucose homeostasis.

MAPK

Mitogen-activated Protein Kinase: A type of protein kinase involved in directing cellular responses to a diverse array of stimuli and regulates cell functions, including proliferation, gene expression, differentiation, mitosis, cell survival and apoptosis.

MCP-1

Monocyte Chemoattractant Protein-1: One of the key chemokines that regulate migration and infiltration of monocytes/macrophages at the sites of inflammation.

MDA

Malondialdehyde: A naturally occurring product of lipid peroxidation. Increased level of MDA is commonly known as a marker of oxidative stress and has been associated with various conditions and pathological states of diseases.

MDR1

Multi-drug Resistance 1: A gene, mutation of which causes sensitivity to a number of drugs and defect in the P-gp production.

MMPs

Matrix Metalloproteinases: A group of enzymes that is responsible for the degradation of most extracellular matrix proteins during organogenesis, growth and normal tissue turnover.

MNT

Micronucleus Test: A test used in toxicological screening for potential genotoxic compounds. The assay is one of the most successful and reliable assays for genotoxic carcinogens.

MPTP

1-Methyl-4-Phenyl-1,2,3,6-Tetrahydropyridine: A prodrug to the neurotoxin MPP+, which causes permanent symptoms of Parkinson's disease. It has been used to study disease models in various animal studies.

MRP1

Multidrug Resistance Protein 1: A member of the ATP-binding cassette (ABC) superfamily of transmembrane transporters that play an important role in the extrusion of drugs from the cell and its overexpression can be a cause of failure of anticancer and antimicrobial chemotherapy.

NF-κB

Nuclear Factor-kappa B: A protein complex that is involved in cellular responses to various stimuli, such as stress, cytokines, free radicals, heavy metals, ultraviolet irradiation and bacterial or viral antigens.

GLOSSARY

NMR

Nuclear Magnetic Resonance: A research technique that exploits the magnetic properties of certain atomic nuclei. This type of spectroscopy determines the physical and chemical properties of atoms or the molecules.

NOAEL

No Observed Adverse Effect Level: It denotes the level of exposure of an organism, found by experiment or observation, at which there is no biologically or statistically significant increase in the frequency or severity of any adverse effects in the exposed population when compared to its appropriate control.

NPC1L1

Niemann-Pick C1-like 1: A polytopic transmembrane protein localized at the apical membrane of enterocytes and the canalicular membrane of hepatocytes. It acts as a sterol transporter to mediate intestinal cholesterol absorption and counterbalances hepatobiliary cholesterol excretion.

NSAIDs

Non-steroidal Anti-inflammatory Drugs: A drug class that groups together drugs that provide analgesic (pain-killing) and antipyretic (fever-reducing) effects, and, in higher doses, anti-inflammatory effects.

pCPA

para-Chlorophenylalanine: A selective and irreversible inhibitor of tryptophan hydroxylase, a rate-limiting enzyme in the biosynthesis of serotonin. It is used in scientific research in humans and animals to investigate the effects of serotonin depletion.

PGE2

Prostaglandin E2: A principal mediator of inflammation in diseases, such as rheumatoid arthritis and osteoarthritis.

P-gp

P-glycoprotein: The most extensively studied ATP-binding cassette (ABC) transporter, which acts as a biological barrier by eliminating toxins and xenobiotics out of cells and also plays a significant role in absorption and disposition of various drugs and nutrients.

pKa

Acid Dissociation Constant: It is the negative base-10 logarithm of the acid dissociation constant of a solution.

PKA

Protein Kinase A: A family of enzymes, whose activity is dependent on cellular levels of cyclic AMP. It regulates several functions in the cell, including regulation of glycogen, sugar and lipid metabolism.

PPARs

Peroxisome Proliferator-activated Receptors: A group of nuclear receptors that play essential roles in the regulation of cellular differentiation, development and metabolism (carbohydrate, lipid, protein) and tumorigenesis.

GLOSSARY

PPD

Protopanaxadiol: An organic compound characterizing a group of ginsenosides. It is found in ginseng and has a wide range of pharmacological activities.

PPT

Protopanaxatriol: An organic compound characterizing a group of ginsenosides found in the root of ginseng.

PTZ

Pentylentetrazole: A drug formerly used as a circulatory and respiratory stimulant. It is used experimentally to study seizure phenomena in animals and to identify drugs/agents that may control seizure susceptibility.

PXR

Pregnane X Receptor: A nuclear receptor, which is primarily involved in the defense mechanism against foreign toxic substances as well as upregulation of the expression of proteins involved in the detoxification and clearance of such products from the body.

QA

Quinolinic Acid: An endogenous metabolite of the kynurenine pathway and a potent neurotoxin involved in many psychiatric disorders, including Huntington's disease, neurodegenerative processes in the brain, as well as other disorders.

QUICKI

Quantitative Insulin Sensitivity Check Index: A method used to determine fasting blood glucose and plasma insulin levels.

R_f

Retardation Factor (Retention Factor): It is the ratio of time spent in the stationary phase relative to time spent in the mobile phase (basically it is the distance travelled by the compound divided by the distance travelled by the solvent).

RNA

Ribonucleic acid: A polymeric molecule essential in various biological roles in coding, decoding, regulation and expression of genes.

ROS

Reactive Oxygen Species: A phrase used to describe a number of reactive molecules and free radicals derived from molecular oxygen. They are known to cause a number of deleterious events.

RQ

Respiratory Quotient: It is the ratio of the volume of carbon dioxide evolved to that of oxygen consumed by an organism, tissue or cell in a given time.

RT-qPCR

Quantitative Reverse Transcription Polymerase Chain Reaction: A laboratory technique of molecular biology based on the polymerase chain reaction (PCR). It monitors the amplification of a targeted DNA molecule during the PCR.

SD

Sprague Dawley: An albino outbred rat strain with an elongated head and a tail that is longer than its body. Used in virtually all disciplines of biomedical research, including toxicology and pharmacology.

GLOSSARY

Se-Methyl-L-Selenocysteine (MSC):
A naturally occurring seleno-amino acid that is synthesized by plants, such as garlic, onion and broccoli. It has shown cancer chemopreventive activity against several types of cancer.

SOD
Superoxide Dismutase: An enzyme that repairs cells and reduces the damage done to them by superoxide, the most common free radical in the body.

SREBP2
Sterol Response Element-Binding Protein 2: A protein that controls cholesterol homeostasis by stimulating transcription of sterol-regulated genes.

SRX
Super-relaxed State: One of the two resting states of skeletal muscle myosin, wherein it is bound to the core of the thick filament with a highly inhibited ATPase activity.

STAT3
Signal Transducer and Activator of Transcription 3: A member of the STAT protein family of cytoplasmic transcription factors that contribute to signal transduction by cytokines, hormones and growth factors.

SULT
A super gene family of enzymes that catalyze the sulfate conjugation of most xenobiotics, brugs and small endogenous substrates. This process is considered a detoxification pathway leading to more water-soluble products and thereby aiding their excretion via the kidneys or bile.

$t_{1/2}$
Half-life: The period of time required for the concentration or amount of drug in the body to be reduced by one-half.

TBARS
Thiobarbituric Acid Reactive Substances: A biproduct of lipid peroxidation, often considered as index of oxidative stress.

TG
Triglyceride: An ester derived from glycerol and three fatty acids. An elevated triglyceride level increases the risk of heart disease.

T_{max}
Time of Maximum Concentration Observed: The time after administration of a drug when the maximum plasma concentration is reached; when the rate of absorption equals the rate of elimination.

TMS
Tetramethylsilane: A organosilicon compound used as an internal standard for calibrating chemical shift for ^{1}H, ^{13}C and ^{29}Si NMR spectroscopy in organic solvents (where TMS is soluble).

TNBC
Triple-negative Breast Cancer: A heterogeneous group of breast cancers, wherein genes for estrogen receptor, progesterone receptor or Her2/neu does not get expressed.

GLOSSARY

TNF
Tumor Necrosis Factor: A cell signaling protein (cytokine) involved in systemic inflammation and is one of the cytokines that make up the acute phase reaction. The primary role of TNF is regulation of immune cells.

TRAIL
TNF-related Apoptosis-inducing Ligand: A protein with anti-tumor potential functioning as a ligand that induces the process of cell death called apoptosis.

TRAP
Tartrate-Resistant Acid Phosphatase: A histochemical marker of osteoclasts with several biological processes, including skeletal development, collagen synthesis and degradation.

TRPV1
Transient Receptor Potential Vanilloid Receptor 1: A thermoreceptor involved in detection and regulation of body temperature. In addition, TRPV1 provides a sensation of scalding heat and pain (nociception).

UDPGA
UDP-glucuronic acid: A nucleoside diphosphate sugar, an essential substrate for biosynthesis of several important glycoconjugates and serves as a source of glucuronic acid.

UDP-GDH
UDP-glucose dehydrogenase cytosolic enzyme: The enzyme responsible for generating the activated nucleotide sugar from UDP-glucose.

UGT
UDP-glucuronosyltransferase: A cytosolic enzyme, comprising a superfamily of key proteins that catalyze the glucuronidation reaction, one of the major phase II drug-metabolizing reactions, on a wide range of structurally diverse endogenous and exogenous chemicals.

VEGF
Vascular Endothelial Growth Factor: A signal protein produced by cells that stimulates vasculogenesis and angiogenesis.

WAT
White Adipose Tissue: A type of adipose tissue found in mammals. Its primary function is energy storage and to release fatty acids when fuel is required.